# Cure
# Tooth
# Decay

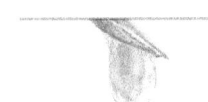

# Cure
# Tooth
# Decay

## REMINERALIZE CAVITIES
## & REPAIR YOUR TEETH
## NATURALLY WITH GOOD FOOD

# RAMIEL NAGEL

### Foreword by Timothy Gallagher, D.D.S.
#### President, Holistic Dental Association

Golden Child Publishing • Los Gatos, CA

## Author's Disclaimer

This material has been created solely for educational purposes. The author and publisher are not engaged in providing medical advice or services. The author and publisher provide this information, and the reader accepts it, with the understanding that everything done or tried as a result from reading this book is at his or her own risk. The author and publisher shall have neither liability nor responsibility to any person or entity with respect to any loss, damage or injury caused, or alleged to be caused directly or indirectly by the information contained in this book.

## About the Weston A. Price, DDS photos

These photographs are currently in print as part of the updated edition of the book *Nutrition and Physical Degeneration* published by the Price-Pottenger Nutrition Foundation.

 The use of Weston A. Price, DDS photos is not an endorsement by Price-Pottenger Nutrition Foundation, the copyright holders, for the accuracy of information presented by the author of this book.

 For more information contact The Price-Pottenger Nutrition Foundation, which has owned and protected the documented research of Dr. Price since 1952. Photos and quotations are used with permission from The Price-Pottenger Nutrition Foundation, www.ppnf.org. Contact: info@ppnf.org ; 800-366-3748.

Golden Child Publishing
Post Office Box AG
Los Gatos, CA 95031 U.S.A
goldenchildpublishing.com

ISBN–13: 978-0-9820213-2-3
ISBN–10: 0-9820213-2-1
LCCN: 2008933990
Printed and bound in the United States of America

For media appearance requests for Mr. Nagel contact: pr@curetoothdecay.com

**For wholesale orders contact Golden Child Publishing at: orders@goldenchildpublishing.com**

**To order copies visit: www.curetoothdecay.com**

For suggestions or corrections contact: comments@curetoothdecay.com

Editor: Katherine Czapp
Cover Design: Georgia Morrissey georgi11@optonline.net
Illustrations: Russell Dauterman russelldauterman.com
Interior Design: Janet Robbins, North Wind Design & Production info@northwindpublishing.com

# Contents

## Chapter 3
## Make Your Teeth Strong
## with Fat-Soluble Vitamins

## Chapter 4
## Remineralize Your Teeth
## with Wise Food Choices

## Chapter 9    169

# Your Bite: A Hidden Cause of Cavities, A Fresh Look at Orthodontics and TMJ

# Foreword

*By Dr. Timothy Gallagher*

**We live in stress-filled times** which unfortunately includes rising medical and dental costs. I see people in my practice who have just lost their job or their house. These people turn to modern foods as a mechanism for coping with their stress, and they wind up with tooth decay. I really understand the difficulty of their situations, and I endeavor to do my best to help my patients by teaching them many of the dietary principles outlined in Ramiel Nagel's landmark book, Cure Tooth Decay. Those who follow the principles have a high degree of success in halting their cavities and those who don't come back to me with more and more cavities.

I have been a practicing dentist for over twenty five years. I am a member of the International Academy of Oral Medicine and Toxicology, a member of the American Dental Association, a member of the California Dental Association and a member of the Santa Clara County Dental Society. For many years I was a member of the Biological Dental Association and for the past four years I have served as president of the Holistic Dental Association. Dental health is determined by what we are willing to do for ourselves; it is our responsibility as individuals. Daily food choices we make have a direct effect on the health of our teeth. But so often when we make the wrong choices and our teeth take a turn for the worse we tend to blame genetics, germs, or the aging process rather than the way we live our lives. Accurate information enables us to understand tooth decay's true causes and to make better choices in our quest to consume foods that support the health and longevity of our teeth. Cure Tooth Decay is a treasure-trove of this wisdom as it takes the mystery out of dental health. Here you have a valuable tool for making the best dental health choices. All that remains is your desire to use food correctly!

Not long after I graduated from the University of California San Francisco Dental School I found myself with a very busy and growing dental practice. Then one day my feet went numb. I went to several doctors and had the problem misdiagnosed several times. Finally, a doctor found that I was suffering from acute mercury toxicity. I had to have all of my mercury fillings carefully removed followed by over twenty five intravenous chelations to remove the remaining mercury from my body. From that moment on I had to practice dentistry in a different way. Most of the mercury-free dentists I know became mercury free only after suffering the effects of mercury poisoning themselves. In placing and drilling all of those fillings, dentists are continually exposed to mercury vapors. But the conventional belief, held by most dentists, is that mercury is not problematic, and they continue to say and teach that it is safe. I used to be one of those dentists . . . until I became ill.

Mercury has many effects on the body, it affects the thyroid gland and it is a known neurotoxin. After my sobering experience with mercury toxicity I became involved in several holistic/biological dental organizations where I continued my education of the relationship of the teeth to the rest of the body.

Conventional dentists view the teeth and dental health as unrelated to the rest of the body, so they cannot teach their patients any holistic practices that can help save their teeth. However, your entire body is connected to your mouth. There are meridians, energy channels, and biological pathways such as nerves, veins and arteries that run through your entire body, connecting everything. I hope to see more preservative dentistry or minimally invasive dentistry in the future. In the holistic approach we examine the effects of dental materials on the whole body both chemically and electromagnetically. The end point of a meridian (bioelectrical pathway) is a tooth and what happens to that tooth and related structures can affect the bioelectrical stability of the meridian and all glands and organs associated with that meridian. An infected tooth can therefore also affect a gland at a distant site. An infection or inflammation in the mouth can create a systemic (whole body) inflammation or infection. This whole body inflammation cannot be cleared until the condition of the mouth is addressed first. The immune system, minerals and hormones also interact with the tooth and related structures.

Cure Tooth Decay is an island of clarity in a sea of confusion as it provides you with practical insight into how hormones control the decay process and what you can do to master the process with lifestyle choices. I have observed that when my patients followed the recommendations outlined in this book they created an anabolic drive to rebuild tissue by replenishing and balancing irregular levels of hormones. As a result, they were able to actually stop, prevent and even reverse the deterioration.

Perhaps the greatest strength of Cure Tooth Decay is that so many disciplines are brought together in a comprehensive package. The pioneering works of Drs. Francis Pottenger, Weston Price, and Melvin Page are presented in a way that highlights their convergent messages. Until this book, dentists have had a hard time bringing holistic dentistry concepts together in a way that is both practical and easy for the public to use. Cure Tooth Decay gives the reader a comparative presentation of the different concepts of tooth decay. It embraces new concepts and modern trends together in one elegant text.

Your diet is the key to creating a healthy mouth. There is no other way about it. This is the key issue, and the central theme of Cure Tooth Decay. When people eat too many processed foods, especially sugar and flour products, they wreak havoc on the body. Insulin levels spike, cortisol goes up, and the flow of parotid gland hormone changes, resulting in cavities. When you consume too much sugar, the hormones that control tooth mineralization change for the worse. When you have adequate healthy hormones, the tooth is healthy and is engaged in the process of maintaining and building healthy tooth structure, through the process of mineralization. When you don't have a good diet, your body's ability to repair and maintain healthy teeth and gums is severely limited. And the result is tooth destruction, or demineralization. If you learn one thing from this book, it should be that eating too much processed sugar and flour products upsets the entire hormone system. This not only sets you up for tooth decay or gum disease, but makes your entire body overly acidic. In the acidic state, harmful bacteria and fungi can thrive.

When people are stressed they often crave comfort foods such as sugar and starch (flour products). The metabolism of an individual who craves sugar is generally in a sugar burning, rather than fat burning mode to produce energy. If people stay off the sugar for seven days and consume adequate amounts of the good saturated fats, they lose their cravings for sugar and their tooth problems significantly improve. After they have stabilized and lost their sugar craving they can have only low sugar fruits: green apple, pear, kiwi and berries (no sugar on top!). If you are susceptible to tooth decay, stay away from all sweet fruits; many of them have all been hybridized to make them as sweet as possible. I once stayed away from all fruits for a period of time, then I bit into a Fuji apple—it tasted like candy!

Cure Tooth Decay is nothing short of a lifesaver for people. The protocol in this book is very effective for preventing cavities and mineralizing teeth. Beyond that, I would expect people to experience increased vitality and vibrancy due to the increased intake of nourishing vitamins and minerals.

Cure Tooth Decay is a godsend for people; I cannot say it enough. It helps readers fully understand how modern, devitalized food causes disease. As a dentist, I know that you don't want to spend so much money on your dental care. I am therefore rooting for all of you to change your lifestyles for the better so that you won't have to. The nutritional approach to treating cavities works! This means people will need fewer fillings in their teeth, and they will walk away much happier from their dental visits. There's nothing better than keeping one's original teeth.

Wishing you a happy smile and a satisfying visit to the dentist, with no new cavities!

**Timothy Gallagher D.D.S.**
President, Holistic Dental Association, Sunnyvale, California

# Introduction

**Prepare yourself to be a part of the transformation of dentistry.** By learning to utilize nutritional wisdom to support the health of your teeth and gums, you will become one of a growing number of people who will naturally remineralize and repair existing dental caries as well as prevent future cavities from developing. And that change, that step towards dental health, begins with your next bite of food.

The purpose of this book is to empower you to take full control of your dental health, and to help you create a feeling of safety regarding tooth decay.

*Cure Tooth Decay* is the result of five years of research and trial and error. Many people have reported positive results from applying the highly potent tooth remineralization guidelines in this book. You too can hope to achieve the following:

- avoid root canals by healing your teeth

- stop cavities—sometimes instantaneously

- regrow secondary dentin

- form new tooth enamel

- avoid or minimize gum loss

- heal and repair tooth infections

- only use dental treatments when medically necessary

- save your mouth from thousands of dollars of unneeded dental procedures

- increase your overall health and vitality.

## 100% Real Dental Healing Testimonials

### Leroy from Utah

> *I was ready to have the tooth pulled and a dentist told me I needed a root canal. I had no money for either procedure. I was in pain and my cheek had already begun to swell. But after over a month of following the dietary protocols it was hard for me to feel which tooth was bothering me. Thanks a million, Ramiel. Unbelievable.*

## Ms. Steuernol from Alberta, Canada

> *I had several very painful cavities postpartum (after having twins) that kept me up all night in pain and made it so I could barely eat. I could see the decay progressing as well in some of my teeth. After following the advice in this book my tooth pain subsided within 24 hours and no longer hurt at all, my teeth also look nicer and my gums no longer bleed and are a nice pink color. I went to the dentist and there was secondary dentin forming in my decaying teeth (as seen in my x-rays). The dentist was impressed.*

## Mike from Ashland, Oregon

> *The practical advice in this book really seems to be reversing my tooth decay!!! Halleluiah, brother!!! The dentist wanted me to have two major root canals immediately and two other teeth filled. When I asked him if there was anything I could do with nutrition or supplements to get my teeth to heal, he said "maybe you could slow the decay down a little bit" but that essentially the answer was NO.*
>
> *That dental visit was three months ago and my teeth have stopped aching altogether, are way less temperature sensitive, and feel generally stronger.*
>
> *Most of us have been totally disempowered regarding the health of our teeth. This information has changed that for me. I bought the book for $28. What a bargain! The dental work was going to cost well over $4,000.00. Think I'm excited? You will be too if you use this info to take tooth health into your own hands!*

These seemingly amazing results are not miracles, even though to the individual it can feel like it. These results come from understanding and abiding by our bodies' biochemical and physiological laws for building healthy teeth and bones.

These rules are not mine. They belong to Nature. I have synthesized these natural laws from my own experiences of trial and error along with lifetimes of research by some of the world's most influential dentists and health researchers, many of whom have been forgotten by history. These include dentists Weston Price and Melvin Page, and Professors Edward and May Mellanby. What I admire so much about these researchers is that they don't just propose theories; they have each spent dozens of years treating and preventing people's cavities successfully with diet. Furthermore, *Cure Tooth Decay* synthesizes published but forgotten research from dozens of dentists, scientists and researchers to help you overcome the problem of dental decay.

## Pioneering Tooth Cavity Remineralization

In my younger years, I never spent much time thinking about teeth. More recently I assumed that my good diet would keep me free from cavities for my entire life. Yet the glass of my limited beliefs was shattered the day my spouse and I observed that our one-year-old daughter had a small, light-brown spot on the top of her front tooth. I wasn't sure if this spot was a cavity or not.

Days, weeks, and then months went by. To our horror, the spot continued to grow and other teeth also began discoloring. As a natural-healthcare-oriented parent, who protects my daughter from chemical exposure in the forms of processed junk foods and western drugs, I was extremely concerned at the thought of taking my precious little girl to a dentist for drilling and filling. Can you imagine what a dental treatment would be like for a toddler? A one-and-a-half-year-old child cannot sit still for a dentist and would not be able to understand the ordeal she was being put through. The typical dental treatment prescribed for young children with many cavities involves surgery under general anesthesia.

Since I wished to avoid traumatic anesthesia and surgery for my daughter as well as the option of having her teeth pulled, I was left with a grave dilemma. I had to decide whether to subject her to a dental treatment—which to me was inappropriately forceful for a small child who was not experiencing any pain or suffering—or I had to find the real cause of her cavities and stop them. At the peak of my daughter's tooth decay her teeth disintegrated so rapidly that the first decayed tooth crumbled apart within a period of a few weeks. This caused me and my spouse Michelle much distress, along with feelings of helplessness.

I know what it feels like to have tooth cavities. While my daughter's teeth were decaying, I was diagnosed with four new cavities. I was not prepared to have more synthetic materials added to my already overburdened body. At the same time as the new cavities had been discovered, I was also feeling a great deal of sensitivity on the sides of many of my molars, near the gum lines which wouldn't even be addressed by drilling and filling my four cavities.

Five years after the original decay, my teeth, once sensitive and loose in my mouth feel tight, firm and strong like diamonds without sensitivity. Five years later, my daughter has four new, healthy, cavity-free adult teeth, and her baby teeth have ceased to be a problem. Her decayed teeth have protected themselves. Success is not just my own, it comes to people who follow the principles you will learn in this book. It brings me joy every time a parent writes to inform me that their young child, who had been suffering from tooth decay, has just been spared costly and painful dental surgery, or when I learn of an adult who has saved a tooth from the dentist's drill.

These results were not accomplished by luck, nor by some special product, chemical, or dental treatment, but by food alone. And you will learn here everything you need to know to enjoy the same results.

## Important Considerations before We Begin

Please note there are now two versions of *Cure Tooth Decay* available with identical content. New copies of *Cure Tooth Decay: Heal and Prevent Cavities with Nutrition* (ISBN 9780982021309) will have the same content as *Cure Tooth Decay: Remineralize and Repair Cavities Naturally* (ISBN 9780982021323). I have done this due to logistical and marketing hurdles related to online book retail sales.

Anyone can remineralize their tooth cavities. However for some of us with severe health challenges, I estimate between 1-3% of the readership, there will be added steps necessary that are beyond the scope of this book or my knowledge. For these individuals good food alone cannot create optimal health. If you have a serious or debilitating health problem, some of the advice in this book may not benefit you. I also do not advocate avoiding dentists, but rather advocate that you make choices that feel good to you.

*Chapter 1*

# Dentistry's Inability to Cure Cavities

**Your teeth are not designed to decay!** They were designed to remain strong, resilient and cavity free for your entire life. Why would Nature plan for the failure and pain of disintegrating teeth? Without healthy teeth and gums, we cannot digest food properly and we eventually will not thrive. In this book you will learn that tooth decay is not a result of Nature's failure or a "fact" of aging, but due to the human error of poor food selection.

Decaying teeth can be a scary and painful process. When in a state of fear and panic, we tend to disregard the most sensible decision we could make: to search for the real cause, rather than succumb to the easy and passive response of allowing a dentist to "fix" the problem for us. Yet when searching for the real cause of tooth decay, many people get lost in a maze of misleading information. Your search is over; herein you will find real and natural solutions to tooth decay.

We have been taught, for the most part, that tooth decay is as inevitable as death and taxes, and that we have no choice in the matter. In this chapter you will learn how the power to cure cavities is in your hands. We will examine the history of dentistry so that you can become aware of how false and misleading beliefs about tooth decay can turn you into a dentistry victim.

## *Reaffirm Your Choice to Cure Your Cavities*

Change begins with a decision. By picking up this book you have either made the decision already, or are considering an important decision in your life: the decision to be responsible for your teeth in a new way. For those who have decided "I want to cure my own cavities," I want to affirm to you that this is an enlivening decision to make. For those of you who have yet to decide, I urge you to look deeply within for a moment and see if you are willing to commit to do what it takes to change the fate of your teeth.

The essential keys to remineralizing teeth are found not only in this book. The answers are within your biology but they simply have been lost or misplaced. This is a guidebook designed to help you establish and implement your own tooth or gum healing diet and to restore a connection with your body through food.

You are not a passive victim to tooth decay. Rather by mistake, you have likely contributed to your teeth's own demise. This principal of personal respon-

1

sibility brings us self-respect, integrity, and a sense of hope that what seems to be outside of our realm is actually under our personal control. I have found that healing cavities is not just about the physical process of substituting nutrient-devoid foods for their nutrient-rich alternatives. It is an opening up to life itself. It is reaching out and growing. It is a small death of the old ways of being. Those who have successfully conquered their tooth decay have embraced the principles of this book and have *taken it upon themselves to heal.* They looked within, trusted themselves, and in some ways acted out of the involuntary consciousness that instructs and guides us. Many people are faced with difficult choices about their teeth in shades of gray. I have found that the answer to these dilemmas, whether concerning your teeth or other matters, bubble forth from within you. I encourage you to take everything I have written in this book as a pointer to your inner knowing and not as a replacement for it. You are the ultimate authority when it comes to your dental health.

. . . . . . . . . . . . . . . . . . . . . . . . . . . . . . . . . . . . . . . . . . . . . . . . .

### The Real Cause of Cavities

The essential causes of tooth decay have been known to the modern world for approximately eighty years. Harvard Professor Earnest Hooton clearly and succinctly summarized the problem: "It is store food that has given us store teeth."

. . . . . . . . . . . . . . . . . . . . . . . . . . . . . . . . . . . . . . . . . . . . . . . . .

## Remembering Your Connection

Healing cavities is about being connected to life. Our modern society generally exists in a fragmented state of disconnection. When we are out of touch with life, or out of touch with ourselves, the connection between the cause of disease and its effects is lost and we can feel like powerless victims of disease, without any real recourse. Since modern society is based upon supporting our disconnection from ourselves and others, it has not been able to support a real cure for cavities. Healing cavities is about reconnecting with yourself, and Nature, through correct food choices.

## *Fear of the Dentist*

Many people are afraid of the dentist and there is a good reason why. Their bodies are giving them a strong message, through the feelings of fear and avoidance. "Do not drill another hole in my teeth!"

## How Conventional Dentistry Works

When you go to the dentist for a checkup he (or she) will use x-rays, a dental examiner, and visual inspection to see if there are any cavities present. When a cavity is found, the dentist gives you the bad news. As they are taught in dental school and legally required to do, dentists offer their patients a surgical treatment for the disease of dental caries in the form of removing the diseased part of the tooth by drilling and replacing it with a synthetic material.

## Tooth Drilling

In the drilling procedure conventional dentists will use a high speed drill, because it saves time, which drills as fast as 350,000 rotations per minute. High speed drilling creates high friction and raises the temperature of the tooth nerve causing irreversible nerve damage in 60% of cases. In addition, a negative vacuum pressure from the high speed shatters a portion of the fragile microscopic nutrient tubules within each tooth.[1]

In the 1800s dentists originally used gold in a careful way to fill painful teeth with cavities. But gold was too expensive for most people to afford; imagine, for example, paying the equivalent of $10,000 for one filling today. Since dentistry was unaffordable for many people in the 1830s the Crawcour brothers made their way from France to the United States to popularize a low cost gold alternative—Bells putty. With Bells putty, which consisted of a melted silver coin mixed with mercury, they could fill teeth in two minutes, and no drilling was required.[2] While effective in the short term, the mercury was very toxic and many teeth discolored or died[3] not to mention the other side effects that were caused by mercury exposure. Dentists who placed mercury fillings were called quaks (or quacks) after the old Dutch word for a noisy peddler selling mercury-containing "health" potions and salves: *Quacksalber*.

. . . . . . . . . . . . . . . . . . . . . . . . . . . . . . . . . . . . . . . . . . . . .

**Dental Fact**

In 1845 the American Society of Dental Surgeons banned the use of mercury fillings because of health concerns.[4]

. . . . . . . . . . . . . . . . . . . . . . . . . . . . . . . . . . . . . . . . . . . . .

The economics of mercury fillings instead of gold triumphed and the American Society of Dental Surgeons fell apart by 1856. In 1899 the American Dental Association came into existence to promote the use of mercury-laden fillings.[5] In 1896 the fate of our teeth changed forever with the work of dentist G.V. Black. He reformulated mercury fillings making them less toxic and longer lasting. He also developed new drilling protocols which are summarized by the principle of "extension for prevention." In other words, drill a bigger hole (extension) to give more time before the tooth needs to be retreated. This technique, although changed to some degree in modern times, is the foundation of modern dentistry. G.V. Black's "innovations" included drilling away all the discolored tooth structure, and then creating a wedge shape within the tooth in order to place a mercury filling that would remain secure. In plain words, dentists are taught to drill big holes in teeth, because that is what works best with mercury fillings. This procedure became enshrined in the curriculum taught in dental schools, and dentists have been enthusiastically drilling parts of our teeth that are not decayed, or that can remineralize, for the last hundred years. The problem with "extension for prevention" is that we lose healthy tooth structure. A dental student from India wrote to me explaining this dilemma:

> "As a dental student I drill teeth every week. I'd rather say that I have to do this to pass my exams. When I see my patients sitting on the dental chair with their eyes closed, I feel for them as they are losing their tooth structure forever."

## Tooth Filling

Once there is a large hole in your tooth something needs to be put in its place. Alzheimer's disease[6], Lou Gehrig's disease (ALS), Multiple Sclerosis, Parkinson's disease, lupus, and some forms of arthritis all have one thing in common—mercury.[7] Mercury is considered hazardous waste in fluorescent bulbs at the amount of 22 milligrams. A normal mercury filling has approximately 1000 milligrams of mercury. In watching a video teaching mercury filling placement, I saw myself the messy process of installing mercury fillings as hundreds of shreds of hazardous mercury are spread all over the mouth. When a foreign substance, particularly a metal, is implanted in the body, the body can mount an immune system reaction. This toxic substance can cause or contribute to diseases such as those just mentioned. The book *Whole-Body Dentistry* by dentist Mark Breiner describes dental immune reactions in children. For example: one child became sick and unable to walk from mercury fillings and stainless steel (nickel) crowns, and another child developed leukemia from these same dental materials.[8]

It isn't just mercury amalgams that are toxic. While less toxic, white composite fillings made up of ground glass and plastic still cause immune reactions on average in 50% of patients. One of the most popular composite fillings caused negative immune reactions in 90% of those who received them.[9] Conventional dentists do not check filling compatibility with your body. Composites of plastic and glue can contain toxic chemicals like bisphenol A. Modern fillings last on average 5-12 years depending on the material. In the case of amalgam fillings even with all the extra drilling, only 25% will last 8 years or longer.[10] While there are some good composites on the market, with such a short life span, the typical filling is not a long lasting solution for tooth decay.

After the drilling and filling comes our least favorite part—billing. **Drilling, filling, and billing** is the model of conventional dentistry and it is also a business model. The dentist with lots of medical school debt, a family to support, staff to pay and so forth, needs to make a lot of money to stay in business and enjoy a comfortable lifestyle. The more teeth that are drilled and filled, the more money is made. There isn't much incentive in this system for curing and preventing cavities because without the drilling and filling business model it becomes more of a challenge to turn dentistry into a profitable career. Because many alternative dentists are afraid of being sued or losing their license, they don't want to practice dentistry that is beyond the accepted drilling and filling protocol. The incredibly strong profit motive has many dentists blinded by dollar signs. People know most dentists are in business for the money because they can see it and feel it. It is easy for a conventional dentist to get greedy and recommend the least conservative (as in most profitable) approach to treating cavities. As a result, many people have lost faith in dentistry; with each new dentist they try, the profit-motivated dentist continues to fail to put the patient's needs first. Even dentists have lost faith in their profession. Dentist Marvin Schissel wrote a chilling commentary on the shoddy dental work performed by dentists trying to maximize profits called *Dentistry and Its Victims*, and dentist Robert Nara wrote *Money by the Mouthful*, exposing how easy and common it is for dentists to make money by pushing unnecessary dental treatments.

With all the toxic materials put into people's mouths causing immune system responses, the short life span of fillings, the damage caused by high speed drilling, and unnecessarily prescribed filling treatments, the conventional dentist doesn't really offer his patients true health care, or a permanent solution to tooth decay.

## *Micro-organisms*

In ancient times, when people were afflicted with various types of ailments and diseases, they commonly blamed evil spirits. The belief was that the evil spirit had invaded the person's body and then caused disease. If one could placate these spirits or induce them to leave then the disease would be cured.

Many people around the world still maintain this same belief today, except that these evil spirits now have been identified. Dentists, scientists, doctors, and government officials have decided that disease-causing "evil spirits" are now real, in the form of micro-organisms (viruses, bacteria, etc.). The prevalent and accepted theory is that these viruses and bacteria are the basic or primary cause of disease—including tooth decay. This theory of disease, labeled the germ theory, became cemented in our minds thanks to the work of Louis Pasteur (1822–1895) who is famous for the invention of pasteurization. Mr. Pasteur proposed a theory of disease that is now the basis of most forms of modern medicine. This theory projects the idea that pathogenic bacteria exist outside the body and that when our body's defenses are lowered bacteria can invade the body and cause disease. Pasteur's "science" has remained the status quo despite a large body of evidence showing that bacteria don't invade people, but rather that they evolve and change based upon their environment. The effect of Mr. Pasteur's contribution to medical thought has led us to our modern system of dental care in which we attempt to cure cavities by killing the evil invading force-bacteria.

## Conventional Dentistry's Losing Battle Against Bacteria

When disease like tooth decay is our enemy then we must fight it. We create war and thus inner and outer conflicts. Conventional dentistry is engaged in fighting this war. Bacteria are the enemy and your mouth is the battleground. Yet no matter how much money you spend on dentistry, the war against bacteria never seems to be won.

The modern system of dentistry has evolved from the combination of beliefs that tooth decay is caused by bacteria (identified as *Streptococcus mutans*) and the belief that bacteria eat foods in the mouth and produce acid that causes teeth to decay. Dentistry then aims to control bacterial growth in the mouth for treatment and prevention of tooth cavities. Dentistry's war against bacteria can be summarized as follows:

1. You must brush your teeth all the time to eliminate these "disease causing" bacteria.

2. You must rinse your mouth with chemicals to eliminate more "dangerous" bacteria.

3. You must floss to eliminate the remaining bacteria and food particles.

4. When those three tactics do not work, you must pay a dentist to remove the bacterial infestations with drilling.

5. When a dental drill cannot remove the bacteria and the bacterial growth progresses, the tooth root can become infected. This requires a root canal to attempt to clean out the bacteria from within the tooth.

6. Finally, when all those procedures fail to keep your tooth alive from the supposed onslaught of bacterial invaders, the tooth must be removed and a fake tooth or no tooth is what remains.

By the time the sixth stage is reached, even after spending thousands of dollars on dental care, the war is lost. No matter how much money you spend, or how much a dentist drills your teeth, the cure for cavities remains elusive. Modern treatments do limit some pain and suffering, but if the basic cause of tooth decay (your diet) is not addressed, your teeth continue to decay.

## *Dental Alert: Bacteria are Not the Primary Cause of Cavities*

The foundational theory of modern dentistry was synthesized in 1883 by dentist W. D. Miller. He found that extracted teeth immersed in fermenting mixtures of bread and saliva produced what appeared to be tooth decay. He thought that acids in the mouth that were formed by microorganisms dissolved teeth. Yet Dr. Miller himself never believed that tooth decay was caused by bacteria. Rather he believed that bacteria and their acid where a part of the process of decay. Most importantly he believed that a strong tooth would not decay.

Dr. Miller wrote this:

> *The extent to which any tooth suffers from the action of the acid depends upon its density and structure, but more particularly upon the perfection of the enamel and the protection of the neck of the tooth by healthy gums. What we might call the perfect tooth would resist indefinitely the same acid to which a tooth of opposite character would succumb in a few weeks.*[11]

In simple terms, Dr. Miller believed a dense strong tooth would "resist indefinitely" an attack from acid, whether it be from bacteria or from food. Meanwhile, a non-dense tooth would succumb quickly to any sort of acid, from bacteria or otherwise. Dr. Miller also wrote that, "The invasion of the micro-organisms is always preceded by the extraction of lime salts."[12] In plain terms, the tooth loses its mineral density first (lime salts), and then microorganisms can cause trouble.

Over one hundred and twenty years later dentistry and the American Dental Association (ADA) sticks with Dr. Miller's theory while leaving out vital information. They write,

> *[Tooth decay] occurs when foods containing carbohydrates (sugars and starches) such as milk, pop, raisins, cakes or candy are frequently left on the teeth. Bacteria that live in the mouth thrive on these foods, producing acids as a result. Over a period of time, these acids destroy tooth enamel, resulting in tooth decay.*[13]

The difference from Dr. Miller's 1883 theory and dentistry's 2009 theory is that Dr. Miller knew that the tooth's density and structure are what protected it against tooth decay, whereas today, dentists are taught that it is the bacteria by themselves that cause tooth decay. **Other than in how food sticks to teeth, dentists believe that diet has little to do with tooth cavities.**

The modern theory of tooth decay further dissolves because white sugar actually has the ability to incapacitate microorganisms since it attracts water.[14] In a 20% sugar solution, bacteria will perish.[15] Yes, bacteria are present as a result of the process of tooth decay, but a lot of sugar at once will destroy them. If dentistry is correct about bacteria, then a high sugar diet should eliminate them.

Bacteria exist everywhere and are nearly impossible to get rid of completely. More than 400 different bacteria are now associated with dental disease, and many more have yet to be discovered.[16] Since bacteria are a part of life, with some good ones and some bad ones and trillions of them everywhere, dentistry's approach to eliminate bacteria seems hopeless.

In 1922 dentist Percy Howe read before the ADA that his research team tried and failed to reproduce dental decay by feeding and inoculating guinea pigs with various bacteria associated with gum disease and tooth decay. He said, "In no case did we succeed in establishing dental disease by these means."[17] However Dr. Howe had no problems in creating tooth decay in guinea pigs by removing vitamin C from their diet.

That bacteria are the cause of tooth cavities was adopted from Dr. Miller's research but was never proven. In the 1940s at an International Association of Dental Research meeting the debate about the cause of cavities was put to an end. By the power of vote Dr. Miller's acid / bacterial theory was adopted as fact despite contradictory evidence and theories.[18]

The competing theory of the time was called the proteolysis-chelation theory and was proposed by Dr. Albert Schatz. This theory suggested that enzymes (not bacteria) and chelating agents which are common in plants and animals (not acid) were the cause of tooth decay. In Dr. Schatz's proteolysis-chelation theory, it is diet, trace elements, and hormonal balance that are key factors in triggering enzymes and tooth mineral chelation which results in tooth decay.[19]

From 1954 to today, the life work of dentist Ralph Steinman and his colleague Dr. John Leonora give proof that tooth decay is triggered by our bodies' physiology as a result of our diet. The hypothalamus in our brain regulates the relationship between our nervous system and our glandular system through the pituitary gland. Drs. Leonora and Steinman found that the hypothalamus communicates with glands in our jaw called the parotid glands via parotid hormone releasing factor. When the parotid gland is stimulated by the hypothalamus it releases parotid hormone which triggers a movement of mineral rich dental lymph through microscopic channels in our teeth.[20] This mineral-rich fluid cleans teeth and remineralizes them. When a cavity-causing diet is ingested, the hypothalamus stops telling the parotid gland to release the hormone that circulates the dental remineralizing fluid. Over time, this interruption of mineral-rich fluid results in tooth destruction, what we know as tooth decay. That the parotid gland is in charge of tooth remineralization explains to me why a small portion of the population is immune to tooth decay, even with a relatively poor diet. They were born with a strong parotid gland. Dr. Steinman's rat studies showed that while bacteria produce acid, **there is no correlation between acid produced by bacteria and the presence of tooth decay.**[21]

Even in Dr. Miller's often cited 1883 bacterial / acid theory of tooth decay, the strength of the tooth is what makes it immune to cavities. In 1922, bacteria were then proven by Dr. Howe not to cause cavities. In the 1940s the theory of tooth decay was voted upon, but could not be proven by dentists. This vote discarded Dr. Schatz's proteolysis-chelation theory which described an alternative biological method of tooth decay from enzymes and chelating agents. Most recently Dr. Steinman has shown that tooth decay is regulated by our glandular system through hormones which are controlled by diet. From 1883 to today, there is a chain of evidence that supports the premise that it is diet, and not bacteria, which causes cavities. On the essential level of responsibility, if germs cause cavities, then humanity will continue to be the victim to the dreaded plague of tooth decay. Yet when diet is understood as the cause of cavities, we have full control to heal and prevent tooth decay.

## *The Failure of Conventional Dentistry*

As we age, tooth decay becomes more and more prevalent as seen in the "tooth decay over lifespan" chart. As we age we also lose more teeth. Not including wisdom teeth the average 20 to 39-year-old is missing 1 tooth, the average 40 to 59-year-old 3.5 teeth, and those aged 60 and over are missing 8 teeth.

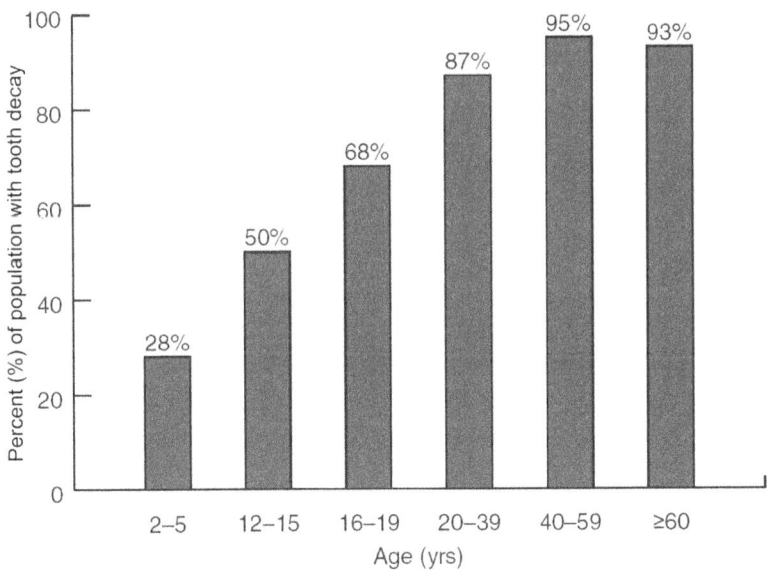

**Tooth Decay over Lifespan**

*National Center for Health Statistics.[23]*

Further tooth decay statistics for people over the age of 40 are dismal. On average, 45.89 per cent of all teeth in this age group have been affected by decay. That average represents nearly half the teeth in each person's mouth having been affected by decay. This situation only gets worse. By the time you reach the age of 60, 62.36 per cent of all teeth have been affected by decay. [22]

While one can argue that the increase of tooth decay with age is due to the inherent break down of the body over time, it doesn't explain why tooth decay is now on the rise among young children. Tooth decay in primary (baby) teeth of children aged 2 to 5 years increased from 24 percent to 28 percent between 1988-1994 and 1999-2004.[24] Along with this increase in decay came an increase in dental treatments. If tooth decay is caused by the aging process, why are more young children suffering from it? And why hasn't the increase in dental treatments in these young children stopped the tooth decay?

. . . . . . . . . . . . . . . . . . . . . . . . . . . . . . . . . . . . . . . . . . . . . . . . . . . . . .

> If dental drilling, root canals, tooth pulling, mass water fluoridation, tooth brushing and toothpastes were the proper treatments for cavities, then we would not see this increase in tooth decay over time.

. . . . . . . . . . . . . . . . . . . . . . . . . . . . . . . . . . . . . . . . . . . . . . . . . . . . . .

Are we to assume that over 90 percent of the population is not following the prescribed protocol? I don't think so. Rather there is something fundamentally wrong with this "modern" war-on-bacteria approach to preventing and treating tooth decay.

*Chapter 2*

# Dentist Weston Price Discovers the Cure

**In 1915 prominent dentist Weston Price** was appointed as the first research director of the National Dental Association. A few years later the association changed its name to The American Dental Association (ADA). In 1936, writing in the *Journal of the American Dental Association* (which is still in publication), Dr. Price painted a picture of tooth decay that was very different from the one we have today. He wrote of people who did not use toothbrushes, yet were immune to tooth decay.

> *All groups having a liberal supply of minerals particularly phosphorus, and a liberal supply of fat-soluble activators, had 100 per cent immunity to dental caries.*[25]

Let's examine some of Dr. Price's fascinating field studies of people immune to tooth decay.

## Lack of Nutrition is the Cause of Physical Degeneration

Dr. Weston Price realized that something was fundamentally wrong with the way we live and set out to explore the world to find out what it was. During the 1930s, Dr. Price was able to document the sharp decline in health experienced by previously healthy people who came into contact with modern civilization. The revealing findings of Dr. Price, published in his book *Nutrition and Physical Degeneration*, along with his telling photographs, bring home the important fact that our modern food and lifestyle are the primary causes of tooth decay.

## The Healthy People of the Loetschental Valley, Switzerland

In 1931 and 1932, Dr. Price traveled to the remote Loetschental Valley in the Swiss Alps. The people of the valley lived in harmony with nature, which resulted in a seemingly peaceful existence. Dr. Price wrote of the superior character and health of these people and the sublime lands of the isolated valleys in the remote Swiss Alps:

**Isolated Swiss Alps Children Were Remarkably Healthy**

© *Price-Pottenger Nutrition Foundation, www.ppnf.org*

*Normal design of face and dental arches when adequate nutrition is provided for both the parents and the children. Note the well developed nostrils.[29] (Original caption.)*

> *They have neither physician nor dentist because they have so little need for them; they have neither policeman nor jail, because they have no need for them.[26]*

This harmony is also evident in the production of food:

> *While the cows spend the warm summer on the verdant knolls and wooded slopes near the glaciers and fields of perpetual snow, they have a period of high and rich productivity of milk…This cheese contains the natural butter fat and minerals of the splendid milk and is a virtual storehouse of life for the coming winter.[27]*

Reverend John Siegen, the pastor of the one church in the valley, told Dr. Price about the divine characteristics of butter and cheese made from the milk of the grazing cows:

## Modern Swiss Children Have Lost Their Health

© Price-Pottenger Nutrition Foundation, www.ppnf.org

*In the modernized districts of Switzerland tooth decay is rampant. The girl, upper left, is sixteen and the one to the right is younger. They use white bread and sweets liberally. The two children below have very badly formed dental arches with crowding of the teeth. This deformity is not due to heredity.*[30] *(Original caption.)*

> *He told me that they recognize the presence of Divinity in the life-giving qualities of the butter made in June when cows have arrived for pasturage near the glaciers. He gathers the people together to thank the kind Father for evidence of his Being in the life-giving qualities of butter and cheese when the cows eat the grass near the snow line... The natives of the valley are able to recognize the superior quality of their June butter, and, without knowing exactly why, pay it due homage.*[28]

It was neither good genes nor luck that kept these isolated Swiss in superb health. Dr. Price continues:

> *One immediately wonders if there is not something in the life-giving vitamins and minerals of the food that builds not only great physical structures within which their souls reside, but builds minds and hearts capable of a higher type of manhood in which the material values of life are made secondary to individual character.[31]*

I want to offer you an opportunity to connect with this once healthy group of people. They are role models for us, for living in health and relative peace. It is this way of being that has become lost in the modern world of convenience and fast food. It is a result of our fall from grace. By sensing and revering the holy nature of food, ancient cultures enjoyed vibrant health. In exchange for their reverence of the life-giving vital force, especially that in the summer milk, the isolated Swiss received health, aliveness, vitality and peace. Unfortunately in today's world, the once profoundly honored cow's milk—unpasteurized and grassfed—which has brought health to people across the globe for thousands of years, is being attacked by our own state and federal governments. This healing food is attacked because as a whole, our culture is disconnected from the vital force of life, and so real food has lost its meaning and value. It even becomes an enemy to be destroyed. When you or your friends and family reconnect with real food, you reconnect with the goodness of life.

## Nutrition of the People in the Loetschental Valley

The native Swiss diet consisted primarily of soured rye bread, summer cheese (consumed in a portion about as large as the slice of bread but not as thick), which was eaten with fresh milk of goats or cows. Meat was eaten once a week and smaller portions of butter, vegetables and barley were consumed regularly. Soup from animal bones was consumed regularly.

### Diet of Healthy Indigenous People in the Swiss Alps[32]

| Calories | Food | Fat-Soluble Vitamins | Calcium | Phosphorus |
|---|---|---|---|---|
| 800 | Rye Bread | Low | 0.07 | 0.46 |
| 400 | Milk | High | 0.68 | 0.53 |
| 400 | Cheese | Very High | 0.84 | 0.62 |
| 100 | Butter | Very High | 0.00 | 0.00 |
| 100 | Barley | Low | 0.00 | 0.03 |
| 100 | Vegetables | Low | 0.06 | 0.08 |
| 100 | Meat | Medium | 0.00 | 0.12 |
| **2000** | | **Very High** | **1.76** | **1.84**[33] |

## Immunity to Tooth Decay

In a study of 4,280 teeth of the children in these high valleys, only 3.4% were found to have been attacked by tooth decay. In the Loetschental Valley 0.3% of all teeth were affected with tooth decay.[34]

# Modern Swiss were Losing Their Health

In the 1930s, tooth decay was a major problem for school children in the modern parts of Switzerland, with 85-100 percent of the population affected. The local health director advised sun tanning for the children as it was believed that the vitamins produced from the sunlight would prevent tooth decay. However, this tactic did not work. The modernized Swiss no longer ate their native diets of soured rye bread, summer cheese, summer butter and fresh goat or cow milk.

## The Nutrition of Modern Swiss

Foods that the modern Swiss ate that promoted tooth decay included white-flour products, marmalades, jams, canned vegetables, confections, and fruits. All of these devitalized foods were transported to the area. Only limited supplies of vegetables were grown locally.

While there are several differences between the modern and isolated diets, there are two points of significant interest. When you compare these two tables, the key nutrient differences between the diets are not related to rye bread vs. white bread. Rather 500 calories of the modern diet comes from sweets and chocolate which are low in fat-soluble vitamins and minerals. These products replaced cheese and milk which where dense sources of fat-soluble vitamins and minerals.

**Nutrient-Displacing, Tooth-Decay-Causing Diet of Modern Swiss[35]**

| Calories | Food | Fat-Soluble Vitamins | Calcium | Phosphorus |
|---|---|---|---|---|
| 1000 | White Bread | Low | 0.11 | 0.35 |
| 400 | Jam, Honey, Sugar, Syrup | Low | 0.05 | 0.08 |
| 100 | Chocolate and Coffee | Low | 0.02 | 0.07 |
| 100 | Milk | High | 0.17 | 0.13 |
| 100 | Canned Vegetables | Low | 0.08 | 0.08 |
| 100 | Meat | Medium | 0.01 | 0.11 |
| 100 | Vegetable Fat | Low | 0.00 | 0.00 |
| 100 | Butter (dairy) | High | 0.00 | 0.00 |
| **2000** | | **Low** | **0.44** | **0.82** |

Here is an interesting observation from Dr. Price of some of the modern Swiss:

> We studied some children here whose parents retained their primitive methods of food selection, and without exception those who were immune to dental caries were eating a distinctly different food from those with high susceptibility to dental caries.[36]

## Immunity to Tooth Decay

Of 2,065 teeth that Dr Price analyzed in one study of modern Swiss, 25.5 per cent had been attacked by dental caries and many teeth had become abscessed (infected).[37] The difference between the modern Swiss and the isolated Swiss, who were highly immune to cavities, is not an enigma. Dr. Price repeated his observations across the world. Let's carefully look at two more examples.

> Stories have long been told of the superb health of the people living in the Islands of the Outer Hebrides.[39]

### The Healthy People of the Outer Hebrides

© Price-Pottenger Nutrition Foundation, www.ppnf.org
*The splendid physical development of the native Gaelic fisher folk is characterized by excellent teeth and well-formed faces.[38] (Original caption.)*

The Outer Hebrides are islands off of the coast of Scotland.

*The basic foods of these islanders are fish and oat products with a little barley. Oat grain is the one cereal that develops fairly readily, and it provides the porridge and oat cakes that in many homes are eaten in some form regularly with each meal. The fishing about the Outer Hebrides is especially favorable, and small seafoods including lobsters, crabs, oysters and clams, are abundant. An important and highly relished article of diet has been baked cod's head stuffed with chopped cod's liver and oatmeal.*[40]

## Immunity to Tooth Decay

On the Isle of Lewis, only 1.3 teeth out of every hundred examined had been attacked by dental caries (1.3%). On the Isle of Harris, just 1.0% of teeth were decayed, and on the Isle of Skye, those living on primitive foods had only 0.7 carious teeth per hundred (0.7%).

# Gaelics on Modern Foods are Losing Their Health

*One of the sad stories of the Isle of Lewis has to do with* **the recent rapid progress of the white plague.** *The younger generation of the modernized part of the Isle of Lewis is not showing the same resistance to tuberculosis as their ancestors.*[41] *(Emphasis added.)*

The pictures of the brothers on the next pages illustrate how it is not genetics that causes physical deterioration. Rather it is a factor of the amount of modern, nutrient-poor processed foods that one eats.

## Nutrition of Modernized Gaelics

*In Stornoway, one could purchase angel food cake, white bread, as snow white as that to be found in any community in the world, many other white-flour products; also, canned marmalades, canned vegetables, sweetened fruit juices, jams, confections of every type filled the store windows and counters.*[45]

## Immunity to Tooth Decay

On the Isle of Lewis, in a count of one hundred individuals appearing to be between the ages of twenty and forty, twenty-five were already wearing artificial teeth. On the Isle of Harris, 32.4% of teeth had been attacked by tooth decay and on the Isle of Skye, 16.3%, or twenty-three times as many teeth as the isolated Gaelics, had been attacked with dental caries.

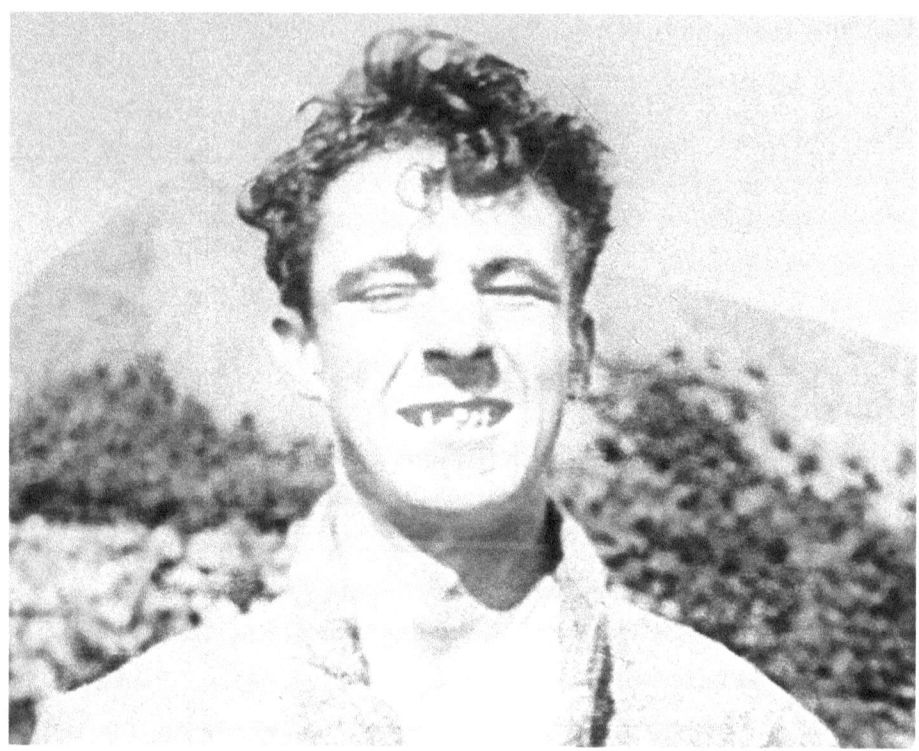

© Price-Pottenger Nutrition Foundation, www.ppnf.org

*The younger boy, seen to the left, had extensive tooth decay. Many teeth were missing including two in the front. He insisted on having white bread, jam, highly sweetened coffee and also sweet chocolates. His father told me with deep concern how difficult it was for this boy to get up in the morning and go to work.*[42]

## Genetics and Tooth Decay

> *A little girl and her grandfather on the Isle of Skye illustrated the change in the two generations. He was the product of the old régime, and about eighty years of age. He was carrying the harvest from the fields on his back when I stopped him to take his picture. He was typical of the stalwart product raised on the native foods. She had the typical expression of the result of modernization after the parents had adopted the modern foods of commerce, and abandoned the oatcake, oatmeal porridge and sea foods.*[46]

> *[The granddaughter] has low immunity to dental caries, contracted nostrils and is a mouth breather. Her grandfather, age 82, has excellent teeth.*[47]

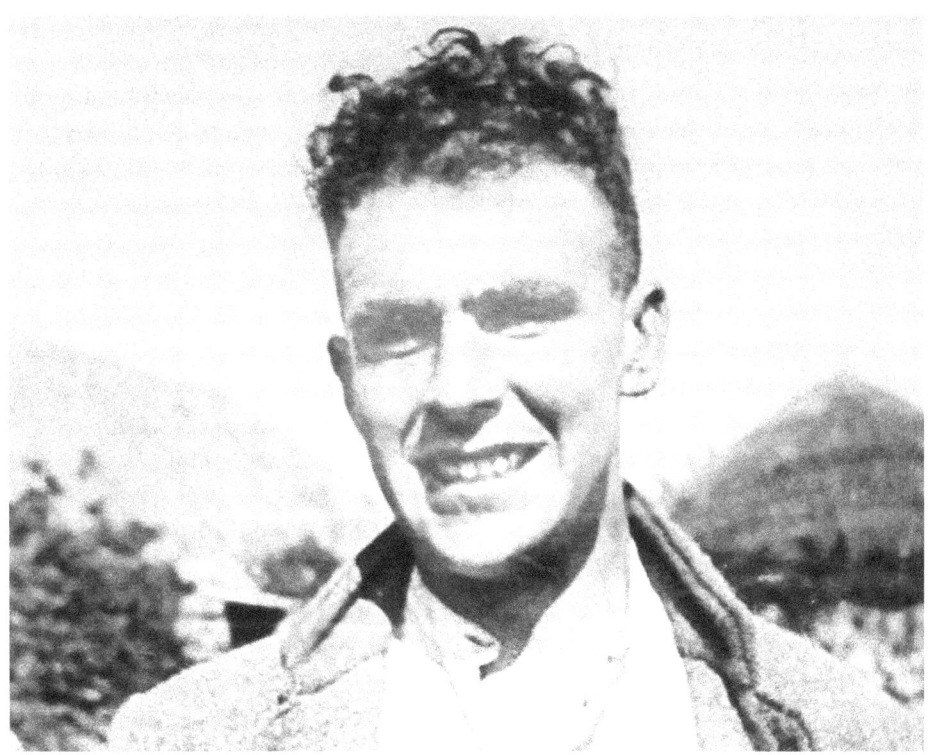

*[The brother on the right] had excellent teeth and [the one on the left] rampant caries. The older boy, [shown here] with excellent teeth, was still enjoying primitive food of oatmeal and oatcake and sea foods with some limited dairy products.*[43] *Note the narrow face and [dental] arch of the younger brother [on the left].*[44]

I have now provided you with two compelling examples of the effect of nutrition on dental health. First, we have the case of the two brothers, one who is immune to cavities and one who is not. The second example is of an older man. One would expect by his age to have a majority of his teeth missing or full of fillings, yet he has healthy, cavity-free teeth. His granddaughter does not have healthy, cavity-free teeth because she does not eat according to the old way.

In both the case of the brothers, and the case of the grandfather and his granddaughter, the difference in their health is not based in their genetics, but in the foods consumed. These observations show obvious cause and effect, yet they defy mainstream medical beliefs. In our modern culture, we are taught to believe that tooth decay and many other diseases are primarily a factor of heredity. I have shown you that this is not always the case. Tens of millions of people go to the dentist and are never told that tooth decay is due to missing vitamins and minerals in their diet.

# The Aborigines of Australia

Dr. Price visited Australia in 1936. He discovered that the average rate of tooth decay among Australia's native Aborigines was zero percent, which means that they had total immunity to tooth decay. In contrast, he found that the average decay rate of all teeth of modern Aborigines, living on reservations and eating modern foods, was 70.9 per cent.[48]

His poetic words paint an important picture:

> *It is doubtful if many places in the world can demonstrate so great a contrast in physical development and perfection of body as that which exists between the primitive Aborigines of Australia who have been the sole arbiters of their fate, and those Aborigines who have been under the influence of the white man. The white man has deprived them of their original habitats and is now feeding them in reservations while using them as laborers in modern industrial pursuits.*

> ***I have seldom, if ever, found whites suffering so tragically*** *from evidence of physical degeneration, as expressed in tooth decay and change in facial form, as are the whites of eastern Australia. This has occurred on the very best of the land that these primitives formerly occupied and becomes at once a monument to the wisdom of the primitive Aborigines and **a signboard of warning to the modern civilization that has supplanted them.**[49] (Emphasis added.)*

Dr. Price explained the importance of nutritious food to our overall health. He observed that the Australian Aborigines, who for thousands of years maintained near-perfect physical forms, have lost their ideal beauty and health with the foods of modernized society.

> *Those individuals, however, who had adopted the foods of the white man, suffered extremely from tooth decay as the whites did. Where they had no opportunity to get native food to combine with the white man's food their condition was desperate and extreme.*

> *[Referring to the figure on opposite page] Note the contrast with the upper right. It is quite impossible to imagine the suffering that these people were compelled to endure due to abscessing teeth resulting from rampant tooth decay. As we had found in some of the modernized islands of the Pacific, we discovered that here, too, **discouragement and a longing for death had taken the place of a joy in living in many.** Few souls in the world have experienced this discouragement and this longing to a greater degree.[51] (Emphasis added.)*

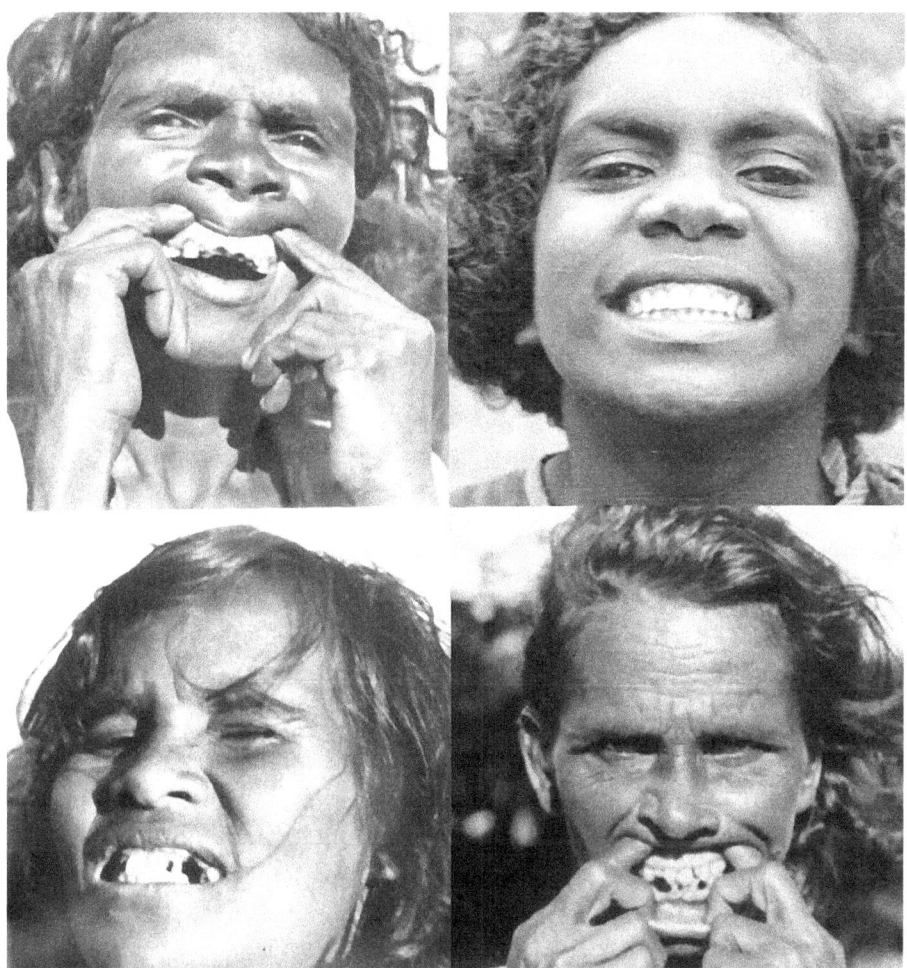

*Wherever the primitive Aborigines have been placed in reservations and fed on the white man's foods of commerce dental caries has become rampant. This destroys their beauty, prevents mastication, and provides infection for seriously injuring their bodies. Note the contrast between the primitive woman in the upper right and the three modernized women.[50] (Original caption.)*

## Diet of Native Aborigines

The Aboriginal diet was a hunter-gatherer diet.

> *For plant foods they used roots, stems, leaves, berries and seeds of grasses and a native pea eaten with tissues of large and small animals. The large animals available are the kangaroo and wallaby.*

*Among the small animals they have a variety of rodents, insects, beetles and grubs, and wherever available various forms of animal life from the rivers and oceans. Birds and birds' eggs are used where available.*[52]

## Modernized Aboriginal Diet

The modernized diet of the Australian Aborigines was very similar to the other modernized diets listed in this book. Imported foods included sugar, flour, packaged milk, tea leaves, and meat in tins.[53]

A dire warning from Dr. Price:

*It should be a matter not only of concern but **deep alarm** that human beings can degenerate physically so rapidly by the use of a certain type of nutrition, particularly the dietary products used so generally by modern civilization.*[54]

# Nutritive Values of Diets Compared

Weston Price performed nutrient analyses of the foods eaten by many of the isolated and modernized groups he studied. In the case of the Swiss, he found that the isolated Swiss diet contained 10 times more fat-soluble vitamins and activators, 4 times more calcium, and 3.7 times more phosphorus than the modern diet. The isolated Gaelics ate 10 times more fat-soluble vitamins, 2.1 times more calcium, and 2.3 times more phosphorus than their modernized counterparts, who lived sometimes just a few miles away. The Aborigines of Australia lived along the eastern coast where they had ample access to seafood. Compared to the modernized food, their native diet contained 4.6 times the calcium, 6.2 times the phosphorus and ten times the amount of fat-soluble vitamins.[55]

**The Dramatic Difference in Dietary Nutrients Discovered by Dr. Price.**

Dr. Price determined that tooth decay in modern civilization is due to a lack of nutrients in our modern diet. Therefore Dr. Price concluded that tooth decay was not genetic but that:

*Tooth decay is not only unnecessary, but an indication of our diver-
gence from Nature's fundamental laws of life and health.*[56]

# Fat-soluble Vitamins and Activators

The components most lacking in our modern diet are the fat-soluble vitamins,
particularly those found in animal fats. By restoring the fat-soluble vitamins to
our diets, we will regain our health and immunity to cavities. Fat-soluble vitamins
are vitamins A, D, E, and K and they are found in fat. Fat-soluble vitamins are
essential for our physical health, not just because they provide nutrients to the
body, but precisely because they are activating substances that help our bodies
utilize the minerals present in our diets.

Dr. Price found that the indigenous groups, which had the highest immunity
to tooth decay, ate daily from at least two of the three following principal fat-
soluble vitamin sources:

- Dairy products from grassfed animals.

- Organs and head meat from fish and shellfish.

- Organs of land animals.

In a rarely reviewed 1936 article from the *Journal of the American Dental Association*, Dr. Price reveals this little known secret for 100% immunity to tooth
decay.

> *On the basis of the fat-soluble activators or vitamin content of the
> foods used, I found that those groups using at least two of the three
> principal vitamin sources had the highest immunity to dental car-
> ies. Those using the lowest amount of fat-soluble activators had
> the greatest amount of dental caries. On this basis, namely, the
> fat-soluble activator content of the diet, those groups using the fat-
> soluble activators in liberal quantity had not more than 0.5 per cent
> of the teeth attacked by dental caries; while those using fat-soluble
> activators less liberally had up to 12 per cent of the teeth attacked
> by dental caries. All groups having a liberal supply of minerals par-
> ticularly phosphorus, and a liberal supply of fat-soluble activators,
> had 100 per cent immunity to dental caries.*[57]

I specifically bring in the *Journal of the American Dental Association* (ADA) quote
because I believe that the public needs to know that what is promoted by the ADA
such as the acid / bacterial theory of cavities and what is taught in dental schools
is contrary to material published in its own journal. I want to criticize the ADA
for ignoring earlier research published in its own journal, by its own former head
of research, Dr. Price. Because the ADA masks this critical information about

insuring immunity to tooth decay through diet, hundreds of millions of people have developed cavities that could have been prevented.

Eggs also count as a special source of fat-soluble vitamins. Most store-bought eggs, however, come from chickens that are solely grain fed, even organic ones. Eggs from grain-fed chickens do not possess enough vitamins and nutrients to merit consideration as a food capable of preventing tooth decay. It is precisely due to the lack of fat-soluble vitamins and activators in the vegan diet that makes it difficult for vegans over time to remain immune to cavities and the effects of physical degeneration.

Insects could be added as a fourth category but this source of nutrition is not heavily utilized in our culture. The "yuck" factor seems to be our biggest obstacle to taking advantage of this category of food. On the other hand, my children love eating grasshoppers, so taste wise, insects can be excellent.

## Why Tooth Decay with Modern Civilization?

Our modern diet rarely utilizes the special foods that isolated indigenous people ate, which made them immune to tooth decay. How often do you eat fish with the heads? Or how often do you eat liver, bone marrow, heart and blood curd? While we do use dairy products in our country, most are of inferior quality, and even can produce poor health due to factory farm practices.

A typical adult needs to eat approximately the following nutrients, daily, to be healthy:

| Calcium | Phosphorus | Vitamin A | Vitamin D | Percent Calories from Fat |
|---|---|---|---|---|
| 1.5 grams | 2 grams | 4,000–20,000 IU | 1,000–4,000 IU | 30-70% |

*Note: never use synthetic vitamins to obtain these nutrients; they are not effective.*

The figures for calcium and phosphorus come from Dr. Price himself. The figures for the vitamins A and D and the calories from fat are based on my analysis of several different interpretations of healthy diets as well as recommendations from the Weston A. Price Foundation. These figures are simply guidelines and may not be suited for all readers. You will need to modify these guidelines depending on your level of health, your weight, and your dietary needs.

Consuming our modern refined diet makes it very difficult for us to meet the minimum standards for nutrient intakes. For example, the US Department of Agriculture Survey found that 65.1% of all adult women and 55.4% of all adult men are below the standard of one gram of calcium intake per day.[58] Without this basic mineral, it is no wonder why tooth decay is so prevalent, affecting close to 90% of our population.

# Weston Price's Tooth Decay Curing Protocol

Ultimately choosing the best diet rests in your hands. I will discuss several protocols for remineralizing tooth decay. But first we will examine Dr. Price's highly effective nutrition protocol.

In a long term experiment with seventeen individuals who had severe tooth decay, the number of teeth with active decay was reduced 250 times using Dr. Price's nutritional program. In this group, approximately half of all teeth had been affected by decay prior to the nutritional program. After the nutritional program, only two new cavities formed in the entire group within a three-year period, which is a recurrence rate of 0.4%.[59] Dr. Price wrote:

> *This form of nutritional control of dental caries is so satisfactory that I can recommend it with confidence as adequate to control well over 95 per cent of dental caries.*[60]

In twenty seven cases of severe tooth decay in children, the diet that follows was sufficient to stop cavities in every case and turn soft cavities hard and glassy. An interesting note about this success is that the home meals of the children were not changed. They continued to eat white bread, vegetable fat, white flour pancakes with syrup and doughnuts fried in vegetable fat.[61] Just one healthy meal a day, as described for growing school children, was sufficient to prevent dental caries from forming.

> *About four ounces of tomato juice or orange juice and a teaspoonful of a mixture of equal parts of a very high vitamin natural cod liver oil and an especially high vitamin butter was given at the beginning of the meal. They then received a bowl containing approximately a pint of a very rich vegetable and meat stew, made largely from bone marrow and fine cuts of tender meat: the meat was usually broiled separately to retain its juice and then chopped very fine and added to the bone marrow meat soup which always contained finely chopped vegetables and plenty of very yellow carrots; for the next course they had cooked fruit, with very little sweetening, and rolls made from freshly ground whole wheat, which were spread with the high-vitamin butter. The wheat for the rolls was ground fresh every day in a motor driven coffee mill. Each child was also given two glasses of fresh whole milk. The menu was varied from day to day, and fish chowder or animal organs substituted the meat stew.*[62]

Another quote from Dr. Price's protocol:

> *The quantity of the mixture of butter oil and cod liver oil required is quite small, half a teaspoonful three times a day with meals is suffi-*

*cient to control wide-spread tooth decay when used with a diet that is low in sugar and starches and high in foods providing the minerals, particularly phosphorus. A teaspoonful a day divided between two or three meals is usually adequate to prevent dental caries and maintain a high immunity; it will also maintain freedom from colds and a high level of health in general. This reinforcement of the fat-soluble vitamins to a menu that is low in starches and sugars, together with the use of bread and cereal grains freshly ground to retain the full content of the embryo or germ, and with milk for growing children and for many adults, and the liberal use of sea foods and organs of animals, produced the result described.[63]*

Guidelines for healing a child with severe tooth decay, rheumatic fever and arthritis:

*The important change that I made in this boy's dietary program was the removal of the white flour products and in their stead the use of freshly cracked or ground wheat and oats used with whole milk to which was added a small amount of specially high vitamin butter produced by cows pasturing on green wheat. Small doses of a high-vitamin, natural cod liver oil were also added.[64]*

*Sugars and sweets and white flour products were eliminated as far as possible. Freshly ground cereals were used for breads and gruels. Bone marrow was included in stews. Liver and a liberal supply of whole milk, green vegetables and fruits were provided. In addition, he was provided with a butter that was very high in vitamins having been produced by cows fed on a rapidly growing green grass. The best source for this is a pasturage of wheat and rye grass.[65]*

## Dr. Price's Protocol Summarized

We will adapt Dr. Price's seminal research with decades of other supportive studies and findings, and then unite the sum to create potent tooth cavity healing programs. I leave you with words from Dr. Price.

*There is a nutritional basis for modern physical, mental and moral degeneration.[66]*

......................................................................

2-3 times daily for a total of 1 to 1½ teaspoons of the mixture:

¼ teaspoon of fermented cod liver oil

*- taken together with -*

¼ teaspoon of high vitamin butter oil

......................................................................

Two+ cups of raw grass fed whole fat milk daily

Bone marrow frequently

Beef and fish stews

Liberal use of sea foods including the organs

Liberal use of organs of land animals especially liver

Lots of green vegetables and some cooked fruit

4 ounces of tomato juice, or orange juice (high in vitamin C) daily

Fine cuts of red meat

Freshly ground whole wheat and/or oats daily * (See note on whole grains. I no longer recommend doing this part of the program.)

## Foods to Avoid

White flour products

Skim milk

Sugar and other sweeteners

*Grains Note: Later in this book I provide a special section on how to properly use grains. Typically whole, freshly ground grains as described in Dr. Price's quotes will contribute to cavities due to grain anti-nutrients or hidden intestinal inflammation such as celiac disease. It's not that grains themselves are poor food choices, but that we must be extra careful in how we prepare and use them. Simply grinding grains fresh is not enough to remove significant amounts of plant toxins like phytic acid. Had Dr. Price known this at the time, his protocol would have been even more effective.

## Chapter 3

# Make Your Teeth Strong with Fat-Soluble Vitamins

**Dentist Melvin Page followed in the footsteps** of Weston Price's findings, and then added the science of blood testing to his research. Dr. Page believed that it requires a 25% imbalance of body chemistry to cause teeth to decay.[67] After 30 years and 40,000 blood tests, Dr. Page discovered the biochemical cause of tooth decay and gum disease: a disturbance in the ratio of calcium to phosphorus in the blood. A ratio of 8.75mg of calcium per 100cc of blood, and 3.5mg of phosphorus per 100cc of blood, with normal blood sugar levels, creates immunity to tooth decay.[68] The healthy blood sugar level is 85 milligrams per 100 cc of blood.[69] When there are blood sugar spikes, minerals like calcium are pulled from our bones. When the amounts of calcium or phosphorus in the blood deviate from these levels, or if they are not in the exact proportion of 2.5 parts calcium to one part phosphorus, minerals are withdrawn from the tooth or other tissues, resulting in tooth decay or gum disease or both.[70] Dr. Page wrote:

· · · · · · · · · · · · · · · · · · · · · · · · · · · · · · · · · · · · · · · · · · · · ·

It takes a continued low level of phosphorus, over a period of several months, to deplete the dentin of its mineral structure.[71]

· · · · · · · · · · · · · · · · · · · · · · · · · · · · · · · · · · · · · · · · · · · · ·

Amazingly Dr. Price also believed that phosphorus was the essential and vital mineral for perfect teeth. Dr. Page's tests reveal the biochemical nature of what we saw in Dr. Price's photographs and observations. The rapid decline in health of native peoples subsisting on a modern diet is chiefly the result of not enough available calcium and phosphorus in the blood. Throughout the rest of this book, I will teach you how to use diet to restore your calcium and phosphorous balance to stop tooth decay.

## *How Teeth Remineralize 101*

Let's look at how are teeth are designed so you can fully understand the process of tooth cavity healing (remineralization) and tooth cavity formation (demineralization). Dentin is the hard, bone-like middle layer of teeth. Enamel is the hard white surface covering your teeth. The root of the tooth is embedded in the jaw. The tooth pulp is in the middle of the tooth. The pulp contains blood vessels, nerves, and cellular elements including tooth building cells. Each tooth has a blood supply and a nerve that travels through the center of the tooth roots into the jaw bone via the mandibular nerve. The mandibular nerve is a branch of the largest cranial nerve in our body, the trigeminal nerve. This nerve connection is what makes toothaches so painful and debilitating. The periodontal ligament lines the root of the tooth. It connects the tooth to the jaw through millions of taut fibers running in different directions. These fibers absorb the shock of chewing, and hold the tooth firmly in place. The cells in the periodontal ligament can degenerate and regenerate. A worn out periodontal ligament is a primary cause of tooth loss.

### Anatomy of a Tooth

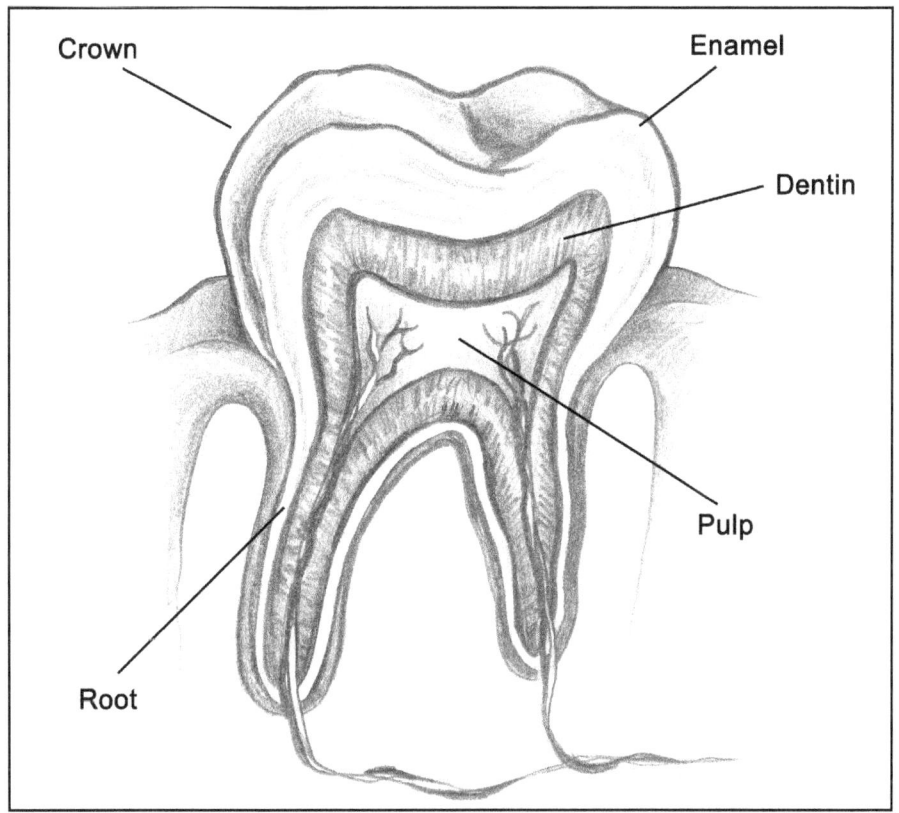

Each tooth contains about three miles of microscopic tubes called dentinal tubules. Dentinal tubules are 1.3—4.5 microns in size.[72] This is close to one thousandth the size of a pinhead. Dentinal tubules are filled with a fluid that is estimated to be similar to the cerebral spinal fluid in the spinal cord and brain.[73] The tooth enamel contains about two percent of this fluid. In addition to the tooth fluid, the tubules can contain parts of tooth growing cells, nerves and connective tissue.[74]

Dentin and enamel are fed from tooth building cells called odontoblasts which transport or diffuse certain nutrients through the dental lymph. Odontoblasts contain microscopic structures that act as pumps. In effect, a healthy tooth cleans itself out. Microscopic droplets of nutrient-rich solution from our blood are pumped through the tiny tubules. In a healthy tooth, the fluid flow from within the pulp moves outward in a pressurized system that protects our teeth from corrosive substances in our mouths.[75]

Dentist Ralph Steinman discovered that our teeth's ability to remineralize is based upon the regulating action of the largest salivary glands, the parotid glands. Located near the inside of our jaw bone, the parotid glands regulate the activity of the nutrient-rich dentinal fluid. The signal to the parotid glands comes from the regulating center of the brain, the hypothalamus. When the tooth fluid flow is reversed due to a signal from the parotid glands (as a result of a poor diet or otherwise), food debris, saliva and other matter are pulled into the tooth through the dentinal tubules. When this happens over time, the pulp becomes inflamed and tooth decay spreads to the enamel. Dr. Steinman identified the loss of certain key minerals in this process of tooth decay. These are **magnesium, copper, iron** and **manganese,** all of which are active in cellular metabolism and necessary for the energy-production that allows the cleansing flow of the fluid through dentin tubules.[76] An interesting note is that phytic acid, an anti-nutrient in grains, nuts, seeds and beans, has the potential to block the absorption of each one of these vital tooth building minerals.

Tooth decay therefore needs to be reclassified to accurately describe what it is. The traditional definition of decay as an infectious bacterially-caused disease is false. Tooth decay really is:

**Odontoporosis**—a decrease in tooth density causing tooth weakness, and

**Odontoclasia**—the absorption and destruction of tooth enamel, dentin and tissue.

## *Hormones and Tooth Decay*

Another hallmark of the work of dentist Melvin Page was the connection between our hormones, glands and tooth decay. Dr. Page found that when our endocrine glands (hormone-secreting glands) were out of balance then people developed tooth decay or gum disease. The research of Dr. Steinman showed us that tooth decay is triggered by a glandular mechanism. It makes sense then that by making our glands healthy we can halt tooth decay.

## The Pituitary Gland

Dr. Page recognized the importance of the functions of the pituitary, known as the master gland, and its two discrete sections, based on the hormones each section produces. These sections are the anterior pituitary and the posterior pituitary. One of the roles of the posterior pituitary gland is to work in conjunction with the pancreas to control blood sugar levels. Blood sugar levels, when chronically out of balance, can often cause tooth decay or gum disease. If the posterior pituitary cannot regulate the blood sugar properly, then this can create a biochemical imbalance that will cause phosphorus to be pulled from the bones. The primary cause of a posterior pituitary deficiency is white sugar.

Gum disease is caused by an overactive anterior pituitary gland. One of the roles of the anterior pituitary gland is to produce growth hormones; this gland is balanced with testosterone or estrogen. The lack of growth hormone production is therefore intimately connected with gum disease.

The posterior pituitary can be brought slowly back to health by eating a diet low in sugar which includes avoiding natural sugars as well.

## The Thyroid Gland

The thyroid is regulated by the anterior pituitary gland. Often the relationship of the thyroid to the pituitary is not considered, leaving thyroid treatments ineffective. A malfunctioning thyroid also plays a role in producing tooth decay and gum disease because the thyroid plays a role in maintaining blood calcium levels. To repair thyroid function, the anterior pituitary gland usually needs attention. People on medications that affect their thyroid can have significant tooth decay problems.

## Sex Glands

Excess testosterone can be linked to inflamed gums and excess levels of phosphorus in the blood stream.[77] Excess estrogen can also cause inflamed gums.

## Balancing Your Glands

The reason for highlighting the role of glands is because prescription drugs, birth control pills, and other toxic or stress factors can significantly influence one or several of our glands leaving us susceptible to tooth decay. Conversely, supporting the health of our glands can support a faster tooth decay recovery. The regulation and balancing of these important glands will support healthy parotid gland function and thus promote tooth remineralization. If you feel that your glands are out of balance, or you are taking prescription drugs that influence your glands, then you will need to seek additional treatments beyond diet. In particular, herbal therapies, glandular supplementation therapies, and traditional medicines like Ayurveda, Tibetan or Chinese medicine including acupuncture can all help strengthen and balance your glands if you can locate an excellent practitioner.

# Cholesterol

Cholesterol is a vital building block for the production of hormones. To have proper hormone function, we need cholesterol. Cholesterol is not a deadly poison, but a substance vital to the cells of all mammals.[78] There is no evidence that too much animal fat and cholesterol in the diet promote atherosclerosis or heart attacks.[79] Many of us are wrongly afraid of eating delicious foods that contain this necessary substance. Do not believe the television, the newspaper, or the doctor who tells you that cholesterol is bad. If cholesterol from animal fats were unhealthy, then why do we desire them so much? Part of this fear-inducing story is the claim that eating too much animal fat raises serum cholesterol and thus increases the chance of heart disease. Your body produces three to four times more cholesterol than you eat. When examined more closely, you will see that cholesterol from healthy fats is not dangerous and that cholesterol levels do not bear any relation to the prevalence of heart disease. For more information and a plethora of evidence, I recommend visiting *The Cholesterol Myths*, by Uffe Ravnskov, MD, PhD, at: **www.ravnskov.nu/cholesterol.htm**

# The Miracle of Vitamin D

Phosphorus, calcium and our hormones all have something in common. They need fat-soluble vitamin D. Fat-soluble vitamin D is considered a hormone rather than a vitamin. Strange as it may sound, our bodies have developed a biological need for hormones.[80] Fat-soluble vitamin D is essential to balance the ratio of calcium and phosphorous in our blood to stop tooth decay.

Professor and physician Edward Mellanby of England is the famous researcher who discovered vitamin D. He and his wife May Mellanby did extensive research on tooth decay which included decades of feeding experiments on animals and humans. He wrote:

> By far the most important factor producing well calcified bones and teeth is vitamin D.[81]

We need fat-soluble vitamins A and D for our cells to produce osteocalcin—the protein responsible for deposition of calcium and phosphorous into our bones.[82] Dr. Price found that modern people suffered from tooth decay because modern diets are severely lacking in fat-soluble vitamins. To cure cavities many people simply need to add these vitamins back into their diets.

## Vitamin D Levels in Foods

| Food [83,84] | Vitamin D Amount I.U. |
| --- | --- |
| Blue Ice™ fermented cod liver oil—full spectrum vitamin D—1 teaspoon[85] | 3500-10000 |
| X-Factor Gold™ high vitamin butter oil— D3 only—1 teaspoon[86] | 1,000-3000 |
| Pig or Cow Blood—1 cup | 4,000 |
| Marlin—3.5 ounces | 1,400 |
| Chum Salmon (Dog, Keta, or Calico)— 3.5 ounces | 1,300 |
| Herring—3.5 ounces | 1,100 |
| Sockeye Salmon—3.5 ounces | 763 |
| Duck Egg—1$\frac{1}{3}$ eggs | 720 |
| Oysters—3.5 ounces of oyster meat | 642 |
| Halibut—3.5 ounces | 600 |
| Grunt and Rainbow Trout 3.5 ounces | 600 |
| Sardine—3.5 ounces | 480 |
| Mackerel—3.5 ounces | 345–440 |
| Pork Lard—1 tablespoon | 140–400 |
| Salmon—3.5 ounces | 360 |
| Canned Sardines—3.5 ounces | 270 |
| Caviar (fish eggs) 3.5 ounces | 232 |
| Shrimp—3.5 ounces | 172 |
| Chicken Egg—2 eggs | 120 |
| Butter—3.5 ounces | 56 |
| Pork Liver—3.5 ounces | 50 |
| Milk—4 cups | 40 |
| Beef Liver—3.5 ounces | 30 |

A review of this vitamin D chart shows a few important points. Seafood is an excellent source of vitamin D. For those who do not have good access to seafood, lard seems to be the densest source of vitamin D. However in feeding trials, bacon fat did not produce the same anti-cavity effect as did suet (beef fat from bovine adipose deposits).[87] Fermented cod liver oil is the most potent source of full spectrum fat-soluble vitamin D. For vegetarians, consuming moderate amounts of butter and chicken eggs will be unlikely to provide adequate fat-soluble vitamin D. However adding Green Pasture's™ butter oil, and free ranging duck eggs would more than likely ensure for plenty of vitamin D.

### Supplements vs. Food

There are many studies warning of adverse health effects of too much fat-soluble vitamins A and D in the diet. Most of these studies are the result of studying vitamins A and D independently and from synthetic supplements, not whole foods. I recommend only food-based forms of these vitamins to be sure the body can metabolize them properly.

# Vital Fat-Soluble Vitamin A

Water-soluble nutrients called carotenes are not true vitamin A. Carotenes are found in foods like carrots, squash, and green vegetables. Fat-soluble vitamin A is retinol and is only found in animal fats. When we are healthy our bodies can make the difficult conversion of carotenes into retinol. Depending on the fat-soluble vitamin A status in your body you made need to consume 10-20 times more carotenes to create the same amount of true vitamin A.[88]

Vitamin A is a family of fat-soluble compounds that plays an important role in vision, bone growth, reproduction, cell division, proper prenatal development and cell differentiation. Vitamin A is important for healthy bones and together with vitamin D stimulates and regulates bone growth. Vitamin A lowers blood serum calcium.[89] This is an indication that vitamin A is helping your body utilize calcium. Vitamin A increases growth factors, which stimulate bones and teeth to grow and repair.

Large doses of vitamin A can be toxic. However any negative effects of vitamin A seem to be blocked when sufficient vitamin D is in the diet.[90] Therefore if you eat a lot of liver from land animals, make sure you are getting plenty of sunlight or vitamin D to prevent vitamin A toxicity.

In examining this list, you will see that liver is the most concentrated source of fat-soluble vitamin A. The magic of liver in relation to healing tooth cavities in part is its high vitamin A content.

### Fat Soluble Vitamin A

| Food[91] | Vitamin A Amount (I.U.) |
|---|---|
| Blue Ice™ fermented cod liver oil—1 teaspoon[92] | 7,500–25,000 |
| Turkey Liver 3.5 ounces | 75,000 |
| Duck Liver 3.5 ounces | 40,000 |
| Beef Liver 3.5 ounces | 35,000 |
| Chicken Liver—3.5 ounces | 13,328 |
| Fish Head / Fish Eyes / Animal Eyes | Very high |
| Eel—3.5 ounces | 3477 |
| Hard Goat Cheese 3.5 ounces | 1745 |
| Soft Goat Cheese 3.5 ounces | 1464 |
| Duck Egg—1 egg | 472 |
| King Salmon 3.5 ounces | 453 |
| Ghee—1 tablespoon | 391 |
| Butter—1 tablespoon | 350 |
| X-Factor Gold™ high vitamin butter oil—1 teaspoon[93] | 200–450 |
| Egg Yolk—1½ yolks | 333 |
| Whole Milk—1 cup | 249 |

## Vitamins A and D from Foods

If you have tooth decay, you are presumably deficient in vitamins A and D. To make up for a deficiency more of these vitamins will be required at the beginning of your dietary change. It is difficult to know without thorough testing and scientific understanding the exact amount of vitamins A and D your body needs. That is why you will have to adjust your dosages of fat-soluble rich foods based upon how you feel. Using Dr. Price's program as a guide, we want at least 2,500 IU's of vitamin D per day, and at least 6,000 IU's of vitamin A. You can obtain these fat-soluble vitamins either from food, from cod liver oil, or from both. First we will look at our food options.

My experience has been that for most people, but not everyone, we are greatly underestimating our needs for these vitamins, so much higher dosages than recommended here might be in order if it feels right to you.[94]

**Three Different Sample Daily Food Groups for Fat-soluble Vitamins A and D**

| | | |
|---|---|---|
| 2 tablespoons of tallow (suet) approx. 500 IU vitamin D | ¾ pound sockeye, king, keta salmon 2616 IU vitamin D | 4 duck eggs 2100 IU vitamin D, 1888 IU vitamin A |
| 3.5 ounces of sockeye salmon 763 IU vitamin D | ½ pound goat cheese 3,600 vitamin A | 1 ounce of chicken liver 3808 IU vitamin A |
| 6 chicken eggs 800 IU vitamin D | 2 tablespoons butter, 750 IU vitamin A | |
| 1 ounce beef liver 10,000 IU vitamin A | | |

Please note that all of these daily suggestions do not focus on the crucial Activator X which will be discussed in a few pages.

# Cod Liver Oil Heals Cavities

When vitamins A and D are taken together they are not toxic.[95] The most potent and easy way to consume the fat-soluble vitamins A and D together is cod liver oil. One teaspoonful of good cod liver oil has the vitamin A equivalent to 5½ quarts of milk, or 1 pound of butter, or 9 eggs.

Dr. Price described an experiment that shows the potency of cod liver oil in remineralizing teeth which was reported in *The New Zealand Dental Journal*. In a group of sixty-six native girls the thirty-three with the best teeth were used as a control group. The remaining thirty-three were given the additional fat-soluble vitamins A and D in the form of two teaspoons of cod liver oil per day. The diet of both the control group and the test group was otherwise the same. In six months' time the group taking cod liver oil was 41.75 per cent more resistant to tooth cavities than the previously more immune control group not taking cod liver oil.[96]

## *The Best Cod Liver Oil*

Recently someone wrote me concerning a miraculous recovery from tooth decay. He had been suffering from a toothache for six months, made two dental visits, received two new fillings on the same tooth yet the toothache continued unabated. The dentist recommended a root canal and a crown to stop the pain. After one serving of cod liver oil, the sufferer's pain completely disappeared and has not returned.

Not all cod liver oils are alike. Cod liver oils purchased at health food stores do not have any of their natural vitamin D intact. Commercial cod liver oil production includes alkali refining, bleaching, winterization which removes saturated fats, and deodorization which removes pesticides but also vitamins A and D.[97] In this process fat-soluble vitamin D is completely destroyed, and fat-soluble vitamin A is mostly destroyed.

The best available cod liver oil in health food stores seems to be Nordic Naturals® Arctic™ Cod Liver Oil without vitamin D added. This product contains no natural fat-soluble vitamin D. If a brand of store-bought cod liver oil has vitamin D on the label, it is highly likely to be artificial vitamin D3 added to the cod liver oil.[98] That the vitamin D is not from the cod liver is not revealed on the labels. Most cod liver oils also have a fractionated form of vitamin E added as a preservative. I have learned of people who developed allergic responses such as warts and headaches to the d-alpha tocopherol preservative added to cod liver oil if they take large dosages. Because of the distillation process, there isn't much of a fishy taste and these cod liver oils are very easy to take. But the key benefit of the cod liver oil to combat tooth decay is the fat-soluble vitamin D, and commercial varieties just don't have it in its natural form.

Green Pasture™ produces the highest quality, most nutrient-dense cod liver oil on the market called Blue Ice™ fermented cod liver oil. It contains all of the cod liver's vitamin D intact because they use a fermentation process rather than a distillation process. The cod liver oil is never heated and it is carefully filtered to keep in all of the natural vitamins. As a result of the fermentation there can be a moderate biting aftertaste, which is not a problem for most people. Green Pasture™ does not heat their product, and the lactic acid fermentation along with the nutrients in the cod liver naturally preserve the oil so there is nothing synthetic in it. I personally use Green Pasture's™ fermented cod liver oil and so does my family including my 2½-year-old daughter. The high quality of fat-soluble vitamins in the fermented oil gives your body the vitamins in the forms it needs them. If you plan on consuming cod liver oil regularly, Green Pasture™ is the safest way to go. To purchase your fermented cod liver oil, go to **www.codliveroilshop.com**

• • • • • • • • • • • • • • • • • • • • • • • • • • • • • • • • • • • • • • • • • • • •

**Cod Liver Oil Dosage**
¼– ½ teaspoon 2-3 times per day for teens and adults for a total
of ½ –1½ teaspoons per day
• • • • • • • • • • • • • • • • • • • • • • • • • • • • • • • • • • • • • • • • • • • •

The amount of cod liver oil you should take depends on your deficiency of fat-soluble vitamins A and D, your weight, your level of sun exposure and your overall health. I suggest starting with this dosage level, and then either increase or decrease your dose depending on what feels best for you. Don't be afraid to skip taking cod liver oil on some days, and to take more on other days. 2½ of Green Pasture's™ cod liver oil capsules equals about a quarter teaspoon.

# *Weston Price's Activator X*

In June, Dr. Price witnessed the natives of the Loetschental Valley "thank the kind Father for evidence of his Being in the life-giving qualities of butter and cheese when the cows eat the grass near the snow line."[99] The evidence of his Being, Weston Price determined, is a hormone similar to vitamin D which he called Activator X. Dr. Price theorized, "There must be some food substance that is not adequately provided in modern nutrition…"[100] He thought this because skeletons of indigenous people show perfect bone growth and immunity to tooth decay. Activator X is this missing nutrient. Activator X is found in its highest concentration in grass-fed dairy, when the animals graze on rapidly growing green grass, and is also present in fish eggs, and the organs and fat of some land animals when they graze on rapidly growing plants.[101]

Activator X likely comes from plant steroids during a period of new growth which are then converted by the animal's body into the tooth-remineralizing force called Activator X.[102] In my experience having grass-fed butter in your diet is essential in order to remineralize tooth decay. The content of Activator X in butter can be seen by its pigment. The period of rapid growth for grass occurs anywhere from May through September, depending on the particular climate. The more yellow and orange the summer butter, the more vitamin rich it likely is. Activator X-rich butter is a factor of the soil, the time of the year, the breed of the animal and the types of grasses, herbs and legumes consumed. Grass-fed butter is not always rich in Activator X, but only rich when there is rapid new growth.

Dr. Price found that Activator X-rich butter could heal rickets and that it brought blood serum calcium and phosphorous ratios towards normal.[103] In practical experiments as well as with lab animals, Dr. Price found that combining cod liver oil with yellow summer butter created a synergistic effect.

### Fat Soluble Activator X

| Food |
| --- |
| X-Factor High Vitamin Butter Oil |
| Raw Butter or Ghee from Grassfed Butter when the animal eats rapidly growing green grass. |
| Raw Cream from dairy animals eating rapidly growing green grass |
| Fish Eggs |

---

### Foods that Highly Likely Contain Activator X

---

The mustard and tomalley (innards) of crab and lobster

Skate Liver Oil

Animal Livers when the animals eat rapidly growing grass

Goose or Duck Liver

Bone Marrow

Animal glands, such as thyroid when they eat rapidly growing grass

Intestines of animals when they eat rapidly growing grass

Small amounts in Grass-fed Cheese from rapidly growing grass

Small amounts in Grass-fed Eggs

Blood from animals consuming rapidly growing grass

---

Without clear tests and scientific studies on Activator X, I could not provide specific figures for these data tables. Besides fish eggs and grass-fed spring or summer butter, there isn't clear data on how effective or potent each food source is in terms of its Activator X content. Where the potency is unclear, I put foods into the highly likely Activator X category. From land animals, the Activator X content is dependent on the season. For sea animals, they likely have moderate amounts of Activator X year round depending on the animal.

I have found summer grass-fed butter to be highly effective in making teeth very hard, and in securing loose teeth in their sockets by strengthening the periodontal ligament.

Green Pasture™ is the only company currently producing X-Factor Gold™ high vitamin butter oil. It is extremely potent in its levels of Activator X and this product is not the same as ghee. As is the case with everything I recommend in this book, it is your decision to use this product or not. It is a very potent and convenient way to ensure you have plenty of Activator X in your diet.

### Activator X Dosage

¼ teaspoon 2–3 times per day of X-factor Gold™ (½–¾ teaspoons daily)

- or -

1 teaspoon 2–3 times per day of spring / summer grass-fed butter
(1–1½ tablespoons daily)

- or -

1 tablespoon of wild caught fish eggs per day

The best butter to use is raw grass-fed butter. Water buffalo, which is used in Africa and India, seems to produce a high Activator X and vitamin D butterfat, but the high nutrient content of this fat could be the result of the animal's skin color, or the food they eat. Raw butter is better than pasteurized because it has more healing effects on the body. If you are using X-Factor Gold™ capsules then 2 capsules are equal to about ¼ teaspoon. The effectiveness of the spring / summer grass-fed butter on healing cavities varies widely depending on what types of grasses the cows eat. Fish eggs may also vary by species in their Activator X content based upon what food the fish eats.

## High Nutrient Butter Sources:

**Local raw butter**—Sources for local butter from grass-fed animals are available at: **www.realmilk.com.** The yellow butter is available from local sources during the spring and summer after the cows eat rapidly growing green grass. You can save high vitamin butter for the winter by freezing it.

**Commercial pasteurized butter**—Pasteurization damages the butter's quality, but it does not destroy activator X. The store brands that seem to contain the highest activator X content are Kerrygold from Ireland and Anchor butter from New Zealand. New Zealand's climate is nirvana for cows, and Anchor is my favorite store brand butter if I cannot obtain raw grass-fed butter. Many health food stores can special order a case of Anchor butter (10 pounds) from their distributor. I recommend the unsalted varieties of these butters. Besides Anchor butter, you may find some smaller brands of grass-fed butters that have a nice yellow color available in your area. These are also a tasty option. For people who are concerned about the fact that the butter is pasteurized, you can convert the butter into ghee. If you are not pleased with your tooth remineralization, i.e., your teeth do not stop decaying on these pasteurized butters, then you will need to try a more potent form of activator X.

**X-Factor Gold™** high vitamin butter oil can be obtained through **www.cod-liveroilshop.com**

**Fish eggs** can be obtained from preservative-free caviar, Japanese food markets, and seasonally from good fish merchants. Where I used to live in Santa Cruz, the local fish warehouse would discard the entire fish carcass of locally caught fish after harvesting the meat. Many of the discarded fish were filled with eggs.

# *More Fat-Soluble Vitamin Sources: Bone Marrow, Brain, Kidneys, and Glands*

This following section is for advanced tooth decay food healing, and is also very useful for international readers. Adding any one of these foods into your diet, even on occasion, will strengthen your body's resilience against cavities. You can stop cavities without the foods in this section or the seafood section if you are taking cod liver oil, or cod liver oil with butter oil. You are not required to eat these foods if you do not want to. I also don't want to downplay the importance of these sacred foods. Learning to love and eat these foods has changed people's lives.

Dr. Price wrote about how Canadian Indians achieved excellent health, teeth and bones:

> *The Indian knows where these special life-giving substances are to be found and he like the wild carnivorous animal is wise in food selection. He accordingly selects the liver, brain, kidneys, and glands. Part of every day's food for the Indians includes eating some of these special tissues. The parents provide these for the children and teach them their special values.*[104]

The Canadian Indians, with their active lifestyle and diet of 3000 calories per day, ate an estimated 400 calories of organ meat and glands daily.[105] For example, it would take about 4 ounces of liver, 4 ounces of kidney, and 4 ounces of intestine together to equal 400 calories. Liver is the most valuable gland for its nutrients and also the most easily obtained. Liver may accumulate toxins, so it is vitally important to acquire liver from the highest quality grass-fed or wild caught animals. If you are further concerned about toxins in your liver, you can soak it in warm water or in milk for a few minutes to a few hours and then discard the liquid.

Eating many different types of glands regularly is a sure way to build your health. Very expensive restaurants know the value of organ meats, and have sweetbreads (the thymus gland), and foie gras (goose or duck liver) regularly on their menu. Including animal glands in your diet will also contribute to your glandular system's balance, because your body can use the hormones in the glands to replenish your own glands. If this all sounds like too much for you, natural hormones can be found in colostrum as well. Colostrum is best if it is immediately used or frozen after milking.

**Bone marrow** is an important secret to reversing tooth decay. Bone marrow adds a valuable factor that helps remineralize tooth dentin and adds a measure of safety to a healthy diet. Within the bone marrow are many important bone-building cells that help rejuvenate the body and promote bone growth. Bone marrow can be eaten raw or cooked. It can be eaten plain, on toast, or in soups.

Organs and glands provide the missing fat-soluble vitamins and cofactors in our modern diet. In many countries across the world, people still consume large amounts of organs and glands. In our modern western culture, this habit has been lost, and as a result our growing boys and girls often develop poor facial structures, due to incomplete bone growth.

. . . . . . . . . . . . . . . . . . . . . . . . . . . . . . . . . . . . . . . . . . . . . . .

**Organ Meat Tip**
Don't forget to eat the brain. For example, in some parts of China children fight over a special treat: who gets to suck the brains out of the chicken's head.

. . . . . . . . . . . . . . . . . . . . . . . . . . . . . . . . . . . . . . . . . . . . . . .

## Organs and Glands Sources:

**Farmer's markets**—I love supporting small farmers. Request your local farmer to save you the organs and glands when he butchers his animals.

**Health food stores**—Generally in the frozen section you will find beef liver and beef or pork bones. Many stores have chicken liver for sale, because it tastes good.

**www.eatwild.com**—This resource can help you to locate local and online grass-fed and free-range animal foods in your area to buy direct from the source.

**www.uswellnessmeats.com**—A high quality mail order supplier of all types of grass-fed foods: chicken, pork, beef, lamb, bison, butter, cheese and seafood (wild, not grass-fed). US Wellness Meats has extended a special offer to readers. Enter coupon code HEALTH15 when you order from them and get 15% off your of your first order weighing less than 40 pounds.

# Organs from the Water

The ideal immunity from tooth decay is obtained when we use foods from at least two of the three special food categories. Butter and organ meats from land animals have been discussed already; now let's look to rivers, lakes and the ocean.

Oysters and clams are exceptional foods. They are usually eaten whole, raw and alive and they include all the primitive organs (fat-soluble vitamins) and are very high in trace minerals. If you can, do not neglect the organs from wild fish, such as the livers. The meat, eyes, and brains, from fish heads contain high amounts of vitamins, which promote overall health.

In many parts of the world, the entire shellfish is valued. In the United States, we crack and clean our crabs and lobsters discarding the most valuable part, the organs and the fat. Yet everywhere else on the planet, every single drop of substance in the lobster or crab is saved and eaten. The shells are even boiled into a delicious broth. The innards of crab and lobster, known as mustard and tomalley respectively, are very rich in bone- building, fat-soluble vitamins. Cray fish, which look like miniature lobsters, also contain these valuable fat-soluble vitamins and are found in lakes and streams. In Western countries the danger from pollution of eating shellfish or their organs is very low due to strict regulations. Shellfish are very sensitive to chemical pollution, and unfortunately we have lost large harvesting areas of our sea foods due to pollution. For example, the destruction of the Long Island Sound lobster habitat was caused from runoff from mass malathion agricultural spraying. I bring this up because when you start to see the value of our animal foods to our health, you also may experience the need to take action to block our own government and corporations from destroying our sea food sources. We can also use our intelligence to restore damaged and polluted eco-systems so that future generations can enjoy the health benefits of fish and shellfish.

Many cultures of the world also know the value of other sea foods, like sea urchin, sea snail, mussels, and other sea forms. People eating these foods tend to have excellent bone development and excellent teeth.

## *Extremely Effective Fermented Skate Liver Oil*

The skate is a cousin of the shark and ratfish, and it looks like a small sting ray. Traditionally in the South Seas, natives would risk their lives to hunt for sharks even though they didn't need to for food. They risked their lives for the oil of the shark liver. To extract the oil they would store the shark liver in the shark's stomach and let it ferment hanging in the warm air for months.[106] Today sharks are an abused species of fish and I would feel concerned about using shark products. Luckily, many unique nutrients found in shark liver oil such as chondroitin, squalene, and alkoxyglycerols are found in the skate. Skate liver is also high in fat-soluble vitamins A and D.

• • • • • • • • • • • • • • • • • • • • • • • • • • • • • • • • • • • • • • • • • • • • •

**Skate Liver Oil Dosage**
⅛–¼ teaspoon 2–3 times per day (¼—¾ teaspoons daily)

• • • • • • • • • • • • • • • • • • • • • • • • • • • • • • • • • • • • • • • • • • • • •

Skate liver oil can be used in replacement of cod liver oil, or with cod liver oil. Adjust your dosage accordingly. Skate liver oil is a hidden secret to obtaining a very high concentration of fat-soluble vitamins, the type of vitamins that make teeth and bones extra hard. I recommend its use along with cod liver oil. To obtain your skate liver oil go to: **www.codliveroilshop.com**

# *Fat-soluble Vitamin Summary*

The miracle of fat-soluble vitamins is that simply returning them to your diet can heal your teeth and aid in healing your gums. The absence of fat-soluble vitamins is the primary cause of tooth cavities in modern civilization. In your daily diet you need Activator X and vitamins A and D. The chief sources of these fat-soluble vitamins are: grass-fed dairy, organs of grass-fed land animals, and the organs and fat of wild sea foods.

By reviewing the fat-soluble vitamin intake recommendations from this chapter, you should be able to come up with your own plan of a healthy diet based upon whatever dietary, logistical or financial constraints you have in your life. I will summarize the guidelines here.

**The simplest and most effective** way to add fat-soluble vitamins to your diet is to use Green Pasture's™ butter oil and fermented cod liver oil daily before or with meals. Green Pasture™ even makes a convenient blend of ¹/3 butter oil and ²/3 cod liver oil called Blue Ice™ royal blend. The teen or adult dosage for the royal blend would be ½ teaspoon or a little bit more two to three times per day with meals (or 7-10 capsules per day, spread throughout the day). The royal blend mixture has a softer aftertaste than the plain fermented cod liver oil so some people prefer this product. Green Pasture's™ products can be purchased at: **www.codliveroilshop.com**

> ### Summary of Ideal Fat-Soluble Vitamin Supplementation
>
> ½ teaspoon of Blue Ice™ royal blend 2-3 times per day
> (1–1 ½ teaspoons daily)
>
> - together with -
>
> ¹/8 teaspoon of Blue Ice™ fermented skate liver oil 2-3 times per day.
> (¼ to ½ teaspoon daily)

If you are financially strapped, I suggest using the Blue Ice™ royal blend in smaller doses. If you must use store foods, then use Anchor pasteurized butter (or Kerrygold) with Nordic Naturals® Arctic™ cod liver oil. **Advanced food enthusiasts use** Green Pasture's™ products as a backup or as a supplement, and obtain their fat-soluble vitamins and activators from regular consumption of a wide range of organ meats, sea foods and raw grass-fed butter.

*Chapter 4*

# Remineralize Your Teeth with Wise Food Choices

**Eating well is about connecting** with what really nourishes you. In this chapter you will learn how to eat to maximize your nutrient absorption and tooth remineralization. In the last chapter you learned that fat-soluble vitamins are essential to remineralize decayed teeth. Now you will learn how to increase the minerals and the fat-soluble nutrient content of your diet. You are going to learn how to replace processed foods with whole foods, and learn ways to prepare food that will help ensure its optimal nutrient absorption.

Cavities in our teeth appear for a reason. And people with cavities have frequent food habits that create cavities. The problem is most people do not know which foods cause the cavities, so it seems like cavities strike them out of nowhere. Even within the framework of the entrenched bacterial theory of tooth decay, the dental establishment acknowledges that the root of tooth decay lies in what foods are eaten. The convenient difference between what conventional dentistry focuses on and what we are looking at here is that dentistry points to foods your bacteria might be feeding off of, rather than to what foods you are feeding your bacteria. Tooth decay comes from eating foods that are harmful to your body. So tooth decay is a specific biological reaction to a set of environmental factors. It is not a random or mistaken occurrence. This chapter will illustrate what these harmful foods are. Many of us typically consume as a staple certain foods that harm our teeth, without knowing it. Pay particular attention to your consistent food habits since one or more of them may be the cause of your misery. Sometimes just removing the tooth-decay- promoting foods will make decayed soft teeth hard as stone again.

## *The Town without a Toothache*

Hereford, Texas became known as the "Town without a Toothache" in 1942 due to the pioneering work of dentist George Heard and author of *Man Versus Toothache*. Dr. Heard explains the town's secret:

> *After a newcomer has lived in Hereford a few years, provided he had drunk lots of raw whole milk, he develops resistance to tooth decay. Even the tooth cavities which he brings with him when he comes to Hereford will be glazed over, if he has drunk raw milk.*

*For years I made inquiry of my patients as to their milk habits. Almost invariably I found that the possessor of a mouth full of sound teeth had been a consistent milk drinker from early childhood. A surprisingly large number liked either buttermilk, clabber or both. The significant fact is that the milk those patients drank came from cows that had grazed on native grass in Deaf Smith County pastures. In winter, as a rule, the cows had grazed on green wheat.*[107]

*My fellow dentists heard me out of respectful attention. One dentist Dr. Young remarked: "If all our patients adhered to Dr. Heard's ideas, we would be minus patients."*[108]

There are not words to explain the supreme value of raw grass-fed milk in all its forms. High quality raw milk will substantially contribute to your health and well-being, and to your children's health and well-being. Milk is very high in the minerals calcium and phosphorus which we know we need for strong teeth and bones. Four cups (one quart) of milk provides about one gram of calcium and one gram of phosphorus per day. This is a significant portion of your daily requirements of the minerals you need for healthy teeth and bones. The fat portion of the milk, the cream, contains small amounts of valuable fat-soluble vitamins like A and D, as well as vitamin C. When pasturing cows eat rapidly growing grass in the time of rapid growth after it rains, there will be moderate amounts of bone hardening Activator X in the milk. It is worth noting that the soils of Deaf Smith County, Texas were extremely high in the mineral phosphorous.

Dr. Heard's years of observations show that people drinking one quart (four cups) of excellent grass-fed milk per day will be immune to cavities. He also advised to take some of the milk in different forms such as: buttermilk, clabber, cottage cheese, kefir, and yogurt. Several ancient Ayurvedic texts, more than 2,000 years old, describe using milk, yes, raw grass-fed milk, as a cure for literally hundreds of ailments. The most particularly healing milk to the body was identified as buttermilk. Since all milk was cultured in those days (the refrigerator was not yet invented) this would of course be non-pasteurized cultured buttermilk. Milk's healing power lies in its nutrient density and the ease with which our body can digest it.

Before the recent invention of refrigerators, milk was drunk either immediately after milking, known as sweet milk, or it naturally began to sour and was transformed into cheese or yogurt. Probiotics are vital to our health and good digestion. Many forms of soured milk are excellent for obtaining these detoxifying and vitamin-creating bacteria. Having healthy teeth is a result of more than just eating well; it is about absorbing food well. An essential aspect of nutrient absorption is having a diet rich in probiotic, live foods. In addition to a wide spectrum of probiotic bacteria, different forms of soured milk including yogurt contain highly absorbable forms of calcium. Soured milk is also low in milk sugar, known as lactose. Dr. Heard's observation that people who are immune to cavities consume a significant amount of soured milk reveals a vital but little known way to create immunity to tooth decay.

**Let's review some of the life-affirming forms of raw milk.**
**Clabber** is a strong soured yogurt-like milk product produced by allowing milk to sit out in a jar at room temperature.

> **Kefir** (pronounced *keh-FEER*) is produced when milk sits in a jar with kefir grains. This is a symbiotic matrix colony of bacteria and yeast that resemble a cauliflower. Kefir grains can be obtained online, or from friends. At room temperature the kefir grains consume milk sugars and transform raw milk into a potent nutrient-rich cultured beverage. It can be drunk plain or in smoothies. Kefir seeds our intestines with milk-digesting bacteria and aids in cleansing and detoxification of the body. Regular consumption of kefir will increase your vitality and longevity by filling you up with more than 60 probiotic yeasts and bacteria, not to mention the highly digestible forms of minerals in the kefir milk.

> **Whey** is the light yellowish liquid that remains when milk solids are removed from cultured milk. You may have seen it on the top (or at the bottom) of your yogurt container. After milk sours, the liquid portion of the milk can be separated from the solids, leaving you with curds and whey. Whey is an ancient health remedy because of how easy it is to absorb and digest along with its vast probiotic contents. Whey can be obtained from yogurt if you do not have access to raw milk.

> **Butter milk** is the liquid that is left over from the process of churning butter. It has a refreshing sweet and sour taste, and will aid your overall health.

• • • • • • • • • • • • • • • • • • • • • • • • • • • • • • • • • • • • • • • • • • • • • • •

> **Suggested Dairy Intake**
> 2-4 cups of raw dairy per day. Make sure to regularly include any or all of these probiotic milks: kefir, yogurt, clabber, whey and buttermilk.

• • • • • • • • • • • • • • • • • • • • • • • • • • • • • • • • • • • • • • • • • • • • • • •

Dentist George Heard's message for the people:

> Reader, would you like to have my formula for building sound teeth in one line? Well, then, here it is: Drink plenty of pure raw milk every day.[109]

These excellent results were enjoyed by Deaf Smith residents because the cows pastured on Texas's native grasses grown on mineral-rich soil and grazed green wheat in the winter time.

## Deceptive Labeling

Milk laws are backwards these days. Milk laws are controlled at the state level, so the law may be different in your state. Dairy products that are sold in larger chain stores labeled as kefir, buttermilk, cottage cheese, or cream cheese are in fact counterfeit. Because of the laws, real kefir, buttermilk, and cream cheese are banned from our stores. Instead, the products you see have a specific strain of culture added to the milk or cream to create these products. The natural, old-fashioned way to make these products is through natural fermentation without adding enzymes. Store products do not benefit from the natural culturing process and are dramatically inferior. Usually the taste is completely different from what the real food, not available in stores, actually tastes like. Equally, the health benefits from the store-bought products will not be the same, with the possible exception of some superior brands of yogurt.

The problem with store-bought dairy is not just in the culturing process, but also in the quality of the original milk used. Most milk labeled as organic comes from cows that are not raised naturally. Dairy cows, even from supposedly organic dairies, are often confined, and deprived of their natural diet of grasses. Instead, they are fed grains and other inexpensive fodder, including waste grains from distilleries which are not a part of the cow's natural diet. The result of this large scale, profit-driven production is that the grain-fed milk lacks wholesome life-sustaining nutrients. In general people do not do well on grain-fed milk; it is too sweet and nutrient poor. Unless labeled otherwise, you can assume that store-bought milk is completely grain fed, even the organic varieties. Although the ideal of organic milk is that it comes from pasture-fed, free ranging cows, the reality is that very few dairies selling organic milk meet these standards.

## Pasteurization Kills Milk

Many people have learned that milk makes them sick and as a result they avoid it. This is rarely due to the commonly blamed lactose intolerance; it is due to *pasteurization* and grain-fed milk intolerance. Probably pasteurization's worst offense is that it makes the major portion of the calcium contained in raw milk nonabsorbable. Pasteurization came into being to try to clean up dirty milk from "distillery dairies" in the mid 1800s.[110] It was never meant for clean milk from healthy animals on pasture.

In order to absorb calcium from milk, we need the enzyme phosphatase which is naturally present in raw milk. High temperature pasteurization heats milk typically to165 degrees or more, and destroys phosphatase.[111] Significant portions of other vitamins are lost in the pasteurization process as well, in particular the highly important vitamin C. Typically the conventional type of milk that most people drink contains fecal matter, blood, and pus. Commercial milk must then be pasteurized to make it even drinkable. Pasteurization cooks this material. It makes sense that significant portions of the population are going to be allergic to this toxic soup.

Because pasteurization damages the probiotic content of raw milk, pathogenic organisms associated with disease can easily grow in pasteurized milk. When the probiotic organisms are destroyed, pasteurized milk lacks its own protective mechanism against harboring toxins that make people sick. In 2007, three people died from drinking pasteurized milk in Massachusetts. Many times when people get sick from milk, it is assumed that the milk was not pasteurized properly. Again, as with tooth decay, bacteria are always blamed. Toxic foods, sick animals, residues of antibiotics and growth hormones are never considered to be the cause of poisoning from pasteurized milk. Even worse, because milk was pasteurized doctors will automatically eliminate it as a likely source of causing a particular disease. As a result, sickness caused by pasteurized milk is vastly under reported while sickness claimed to be caused by raw milk is vastly over reported. With clean hygienic milking standards healthy raw milk from grass-fed animals will be safer than pasteurized milk.

Homogenized milk renders the milk unusable because it breaks apart the milk's cellular structure. It does so by forcing milk at high pressure through extremely small holes which rupture the milk cells. Do not drink homogenized milk. Many commercial ice creams are made with homogenized milk to give it a creamier texture.

Commercial dairy animals are injected with rBGH (recombinant bovine growth hormone), and they are fed genetically modified grains, which are not a part of their natural diet. Avoid non-organic dairy foods. Consuming pasteurized commercial milk raises the level of nonabsorbable calcium in one's diet.[112]

Avoid powdered milk because it has been heated and the protein structure destroyed. Low-fat milk is not satisfying to drink, but it can be used to make some good cheese.

## Obtaining Raw Milk

Due to laws that assault our personal freedom, liberty and right to choice guaranteed by states and the US Constitution, raw milk can be difficult to obtain. In many states raw milk is harder to get than hard liquor, cigarettes, guns, prescription drugs that have known dangerous side effects, and even marijuana. The term for raw milk where it is illegal to be sold is moo-shine.

www.realmilk.com—One easy way to find raw milk in your vicinity.

www.westonaprice.org/chapters—Get involved with and contact your local Weston A. Price Foundation chapter leader. Many times they can direct you to lesser known cow-share programs and legal direct-from-the-farmer dairy products.

Whole Foods® has a very nice artisan cheese section with many raw milk cheeses. You can tell if a cheese is grass-fed typically by how pungent it is. Grain-fed cheese has a bland or "normal" milk flavor. Grass-fed cheese is flavorful, usually pungent, and sometimes contains hints of a grassy flavor. In cities or more affluent areas, you can often find cheesemongers who will have several varieties of grass-fed raw cheeses, many of which are imported from Europe.

## Non-Dairy Options and Calcium Alternatives

Many people are told that they cannot digest dairy foods, or experience known negative effects from pasteurized milk. Yet for a majority of people these negative effects do not occur when they drink raw grass-fed milk. This is because raw grass-fed milk is a completely different product from pasteurized confinement dairy milk. If raw cow's milk does not work for you, do not be afraid to try some raw milk cheese, or raw sheep, goat or mare's milk. Many people who have problems with raw milk find that soured milk such as kefir works well with their system. Over a period of months, consuming kefir will restore most people's ability to drink raw milk.

The goal for calcium consumption for an adult is somewhere between 1–1½ grams of calcium per day. To obtain adequate dietary calcium without using dairy foods, dentist Melvin Page recommended eating: salmon, oysters, clams, shrimp, other sea-foods, broccoli, beet greens, nuts, beans, cauliflower, figs and olives.[114] Green vegetables that are very high in calcium come from the brassica family and include: broccoli, kale, bok choy, cabbage, mustard and turnip greens. Seaweed is another excellent source of calcium. Other sources of calcium could be taro root, and herbs. If you need to look up the calcium content, or nutrient contents of other foods, I like to use www.nutritiondata.com

For a dairy-free diet, you will need to consume lots and lots of vegetables every day, 1–2 cups of bone broth, and a moderate amount of sea food to get adequate calcium. To obtain one gram of calcium from vegetables, for example, you will need to eat: 7 cups of chopped raw kale, which is about one bunch of kale (and cook that amount), or an entire bunch of collard greens, about 20 ounces cooked, per day. Canned fish with bones is high in calcium, but fresh fish will be much lower because the bones are not consumed.

## Calcium Content in Foods

| Food | Calcium in Milligrams[113] |
|---|---|
| Hard / Soft Cheeses —2 ounces | 404 |
| Canned Sardines with bones —1 can 3.75 ounces | 351 |
| Yogurt, Whole Milk—1 cup | 296 |
| Canned Salmon with bones 3.5 ounces | 277 |
| Whole Milk—1 cup | 276 |
| Cooked Collard Greens 1 cup | 266 |
| Cooked Tahitian Taro Root—1 cup | 204 |
| Cooked Kale—1 cup | 171 |
| Cooked Dandelion Greens—1 cup | 147 |
| Cooked Broccoli—2 cups | 120 |
| Cooked Scallops—3.5 ounces | 115 |
| Herring—3 ounces | 90 |
| Cottage Cheese — ½ cup | 69 |
| Halibut—3 ounces | 50 |
| One Medium Sweet Potato | 40 |
| Shrimp — 3 ounces | 33 |
| Salmon without Bones — 3.5 ounces | 28 |

### Calcium Supplements

Many, but not all calcium supplements contain forms of calcium that are not recognized by your body. Non-absorbable calcium raises blood calcium levels in an unhealthy way which can lead to excess calculus deposits. I do not have any recommendations for calcium supplements even though there may be some good ones on the market. I suggest getting non-dairy calcium from plenty of vegetables and sea food.

# Good Soup Heals Your Teeth

There's nothing like delicious soup that warms your insides. Homemade broths are one of the most potent medicines for tooth decay. In the diet of the people in the Swiss Alps who were largely immune to cavities, soups were served throughout the week.[115] Broth from nourishing soup is made by boiling cartilage-rich bones of chicken, beef, fish, and so on. Good broth is rich in gelatin, and when refrigerated it will gel. Excellent gravy can be made with beef or lamb broth.

Gelatin can help heal and rebuild your digestive tract. It enhances nutrient absorption. Aloe vera and slippery elm gruel can also aid in soothing the intestines. Part of Dr. Price's successful tooth decay controlling protocol was the almost daily use of beef or fish stews. The beef stew was prepared with plenty of bone marrow. The best bone broth for tooth decay reversal is broth made from the carcasses of wild fish. The carcass ideally should have the head, and if it has the organs—even better. This broth is especially potent and rich in minerals. **Instructions for broth are found in the recipe section later in the book.** Healthy cultures around the world know the value of soup made with fish heads. The meat, eyes and brain from the fish are all eaten as they are rich in minerals and fat-soluble vitamins.

· · · · · · · · · · · · · · · · · · · · · · · · · · · · · · · · · · · · · · · · · · · · · · · · · · · · ·

**Suggested Broth Consumption**
1-2 cups of broth per day. Consume it as a tea, in soups, in stews or as gravy.

· · · · · · · · · · · · · · · · · · · · · · · · · · · · · · · · · · · · · · · · · · · · · · · · · · · · ·

# Blood Sugar

An important insight from dentist Melvin Page explains how blood sugar fluctuations can influence tooth decay. In blood chemistry tests, Dr. Page determined that different types of sugar consumption cause different fluctuations in blood sugar levels. When blood sugar fluctuates, the calcium and phosphorus ratios in the blood fluctuate along with it. White sugar produces the most significant blood sugar fluctuations, which last five hours. Fruit sugar produces fewer fluctuations but the blood sugar still remains out of balance for five hours. Honey causes even fewer fluctuations and blood sugar stabilizes after three hours.[116] Blood sugar fluctuations can increase blood calcium. This is because calcium is being pulled from your teeth or your bones depending upon which glands are strong and which glands are weak in your body. The calcium and phosphorous ratios in your blood are negatively affected over time by blood sugar fluctuations. Dr. Page found that the combination of stable blood sugar levels with the correct ratio of calcium and phosphorous in the blood results in immunity to tooth decay.[117]

The longer your blood sugar is out of control, the longer and more significantly the calcium and phosphorus ratios are altered, the higher the likelihood of tooth decay. Regardless of whether the sugar is white sugar or sugar from fruit consumption, it still affects your blood sugar level. If sweet foods, natural or processed, are consumed several times per day, then the alteration in blood sugar will be prolonged and consistent. Over time, this will lead to a consistent alteration of blood calcium and phosphorous levels and likely cause cavities. All sweet foods, no matter how natural, cause blood sugar fluctuations. How much blood sugar fluctuates is related to the intensity of the sweetness. Therefore dates, or dried fruit, may cause significantly more blood sugar fluctuations than a fresh green apple. If sugar is a part of your regular diet, particularly in large amounts, then your blood sugar level never has much time to recover to normal.

While conventional dentistry believes that it is the carbohydrate factor of the food sticking to teeth that causes cavities, in reality it is the changes of the blood chemistry that cause tooth decay from sugar. Conventional dentistry advises patients against frequent snacking. Here the ADA writes, "Frequent snacking on carbohydrate-containing foods can be an invitation to tooth decay."[118] Frequent snacking typically is an invitation for tooth decay, not because snacking itself is bad or wrong, but because of the types of foods most people choose for snacks. Typical snacks could be: fast foods, potato chips, candy bars, "health food" bars, breakfast cereals and flour products of every type. Thus conventional dentistry is partially correct: frequent snacking from sugar-laden convenience foods of commerce produces tooth decay. Dr. Page found that frequent meals containing vegetables, protein and fat are beneficial in controlling blood sugar fluctuations. Conventional dentistry is also incorrect about snacking, because frequent snacking of balancing foods like vegetables, proteins and fats will not cause tooth decay. Tooth decay has more of a connection to the type of food eaten than to the frequency of snacking. Wise food choices containing some protein allow you to snack all day long while inhibiting tooth decay.

## Fruit

Fruit, particularly berries, can add to your health. But too much fruit means too much sugar and that can cause tooth cavities by causing blood sugar fluctuations. Most of the fruit on the store shelves today is hybridized. For example, an ancient apple was a small sour fruit, which probably needed to be cooked to be edible. But hundreds and even thousands of years of cultivation, selection, and hybridization have created apples with high sugar content. While fruit is natural, the high sugar content of most fruits means that many people cannot eat as much fruit as they want and remain healthy. Fruit is not a bad food choice, but many people eat too much. Many people have mistakenly made fruit a staple item of their diets, rather than seeing it as a snack, side dish, or occasional treat.

Fruit is best eaten with fat. Fruit and cream go well together, such as peaches or strawberries and cream. Some fruit goes well with cheese, such as apples or pears. Some people consume excess amounts of very sweet fruits. The sugar in these fruits helps calm hunger by providing rapid energy. But fruit does not give the body sufficient nutrient building blocks like protein. Sweet fruits include oranges, peaches, grapes and bananas. I highly recommend limiting these very sweet fruits when you are trying to keep tooth decay at a minimum. Having cavities is a sign that your blood sugar mechanism is not working optimally, and eating excessive natural sweets will not allow your system to correct itself. Once your cavities are a distant memory, you could safely eat more sweet fruits. For some people, cooking all of their fruit before eating is helpful as it transforms the sugars and can increase digestibility.

**Basic fruit recommendations**: Avoid or greatly limit highly sweet fruits like dates, peaches, pineapples, dried fruit, blueberries and bananas until you do not have tooth decay anymore.

**Intermediate fruit recommendations**: Only have fruit once around the middle of the day such as after lunch. The fruit you do eat should not be too sweet. Examples of less sweet fruits are: sour berries such as raspberries, as well as kiwi, and green apples.

**Advanced fruit recommendations**: If you have bad cavities or want to immediately stop the rapid process of tooth decay, avoid all sweets and fruits completely.

# Sweeteners

The work of dentist Melvin Page and the telling photographs of Weston Price show us the disastrous effects of too much sugar in our diet. The more refined the sugar is, the more it is going to cause your blood sugar to fluctuate. The more extreme the fluctuation, the more disturbed your calcium and phosphorous metabolism will be. Fructose-containing sweeteners or sweeteners labeled as low glycemic may not raise your blood glucose level, but they do raise your blood fructose levels. The end result is an even deeper disturbance in your calcium and phosphorous balance than that caused by white sugar. We already have the challenge of obtaining enough minerals in our diet. The more sweet foods that you eat the less room you will have for mineral- dense foods like vegetables and nuts.

## *Safe Sweeteners in Moderation*

You can use these sweeteners in moderation when you do not have active tooth decay. If you have active tooth decay, and painful or sensitive teeth, then make every effort to temporarily avoid all added sweets. Our current policy at home is to only have sugar from fruit. Once or twice per month for a sweet dish we use unheated honey, grade B organic maple syrup, and pure cane sugar from Heavenly Organics™.

**Unheated honey**—Choose honey that states it is unheated, or never heated, on the label. Bees work very hard to keep their hive at around 93 degrees Fahrenheit. If the hive gets too hot, the bees abandon the hive. I highly recommend only consuming honey that is harvested at or below 93 degrees. Honey that is labeled as "raw" but does not state unheated or never heated may have been heated to much higher temperatures than 93 degrees, and many of the benefits of the honey may be lost. For this reason, honey is not good for cooking. Despite the claims of some manufacturers of honey, honey does not prevent tooth decay. It is however an excellent sweetener.

**Maple Syrup**—Grade B organic maple syrup will have your body saying "yes." Many maple syrups may contain formaldehyde residue even though the practice of using formaldehyde pellets to keep tap holes in trees open is currently forbidden. I have felt sick from a generic brand of organic maple syrup, so choose smaller independent brands that are more likely to be using the best practices.

**Real Cane Sugar**—In ancient Ayurvedic medicine, real sugar such as jaggery is considered a medicine. But most of the sugar available in the store today is far from medicinal. Most varieties are excessively processed. Safe forms of sugar are pure cane juice, extracted yourself from the sugar cane, Heavenly Organics ™ Sugar, or Rapunzel's Rapadura sugar. As far as I know, other sugars labeled raw, organic or anything else are likely to be significantly processed, with the minerals removed. Both cane sugar and maple syrup can be safely used in cooking.

**Stevia** (Use extreme caution)—Stevia is a very sweet herb. You must be extremely careful with its use because it may have other medicinal properties besides its use as a sweetener. The only stevia that is safe to use is the minimally processed fresh herb. The fresh stevia is simply dried and powdered. A stevia concentrate which is a brownish color that simply contains the entire stevia herb in a more potent form should also be safe. There are many sweeteners made from extracting components of the stevia leaf and they are dangerous. Be very careful that you do not mistakenly buy a stevia extract or overly processed product. These extracts of stevia will likely cause significant imbalances to your glandular system. Likewise do not use stevia that is stored in glycerin.

## Refined Sweeteners Can Damage Your Teeth

The simple rule I follow for sweeteners is that if the sweetener you are using is not on the above approved list, and not a sweet whole food like dried fruit, then avoid it. It is important that you understand that many sweeteners that have been recently introduced into the market, particularly to the health food market, are highly processed and deceptively labeled. I have had many people plead with me, "but the label says it is raw, vegan, all natural, and healthy." When large sums of money are potentially to be made, marketers blur the line of reality to in order to sell more products. Just because the label presents a convincing marketing pitch does not mean you should be the next human guinea pig. Healthy sweeteners affect your blood sugar level. That is what sweet foods do. There is nothing healthier about an exotic sounding, imported sweetener than correctly processed cane sugar.

**Evaporated Cane Juice and White Sugar**—The empty calories from sugar provide energy but do not provide nutrients to the body. White sugar will cause blood sugar fluctuations which over time will result in mineral losses from your teeth and bones. Queen Elizabeth the 1st is remembered for her black teeth from excessive sugar consumption. They turned black, but did not have huge painful cavities probably because of her otherwise protective diet rich in fat-soluble nutrients. Processed sugar consumption depletes chromium, zinc, magnesium and manganese.[119] Health food product labels often list organic evaporated cane juice. Do not be fooled by this natural-sounding interpretation; this is simply sugar. Sugar is recognized by the body so it is far better than any of the sugar replacements. If you are going to choose to buy a packaged food that is sweet, you want it to contain either sugar or fruit as a sweetener. That being said, consuming sugar gives us calories that are not nutrient dense. The replacement of nutrient-dense foods with nutrient-poor sugar in our modern diet is in part what has contributed to tooth decay with the rise of modern civilization.

**Xylitol**—A research report in the *Journal of the American Dental Association* suggested that claims that xylitol stops cavities need further studies.[120] Xylitol is a sugar alcohol, and not simply a sugar. Pets can overdose on xylitol, with side effects ranging from seizures to liver damage, and even death. Xylitol does not have what is known as "GRAS" status, or Generally Recognized As Safe for consumption status by the federal government. It is approved as a food additive instead.[121] That is why it is chiefly found in products that are "cosmetic" by legal definition, such as toothpaste or chewing gum.[122] Xylitol is metabolized primarily in the liver.[123] Xylitol's anti-cavity properties are purported to depend on the fact that bacteria cannot digest sugar alcohols and convert them into acids. Yet in chapter one I clearly demonstrated that bacteria and acids are not the primary culprits in tooth decay. Also avoid the other unnatural sounding sugar alcohol sweeteners such as sorbitol, mannitol, maltitol, and erythritol.

**High Fructose Corn Syrup (Corn Sugar)**—This is by far the worst sweetener for our teeth and overall health. What is confusing to people about fructose, is that fructose in manmade products is not the same as fructose in fruit. A synthetic sugar and a natural sugar have been given the same name. Because high fructose corn syrup contains the synthetic form of fructose, it is toxic to the body. This explains why in study after study high fructose corn syrup is linked to serious diseases like pancreatic cancer, diabetes, and obesity.[124] My experience is that consuming foods containing fructose is a recipe for glandular imbalances that lead to severe tooth decay. Avoid high fructose corn syrup like the plague. Manmade fructose is hiding in processed foods under different aliases including: the highly processed fructooligosaccharides (FOS) or inulin as well as fructose, or corn syrup. Sweetened drinks, soft drinks and food bars are just a few of the foods commonly sweetened by fructose. The prevalence of the dangerous high fructose corn syrup in our foods is due to government subsidies to the corn industry which make fructose cheaper than natural sugar. This policy is not a good use of our tax dollars.

· · · · · · · · · · · · · · · · · · · · · · · · · · · · · · · · · · · · · · · · · · · · · ·

### The Double Danger of Soft Drinks

Soft drinks contain tons of sugar and are highly acidic. They rob your body of calcium and magnesium once because of the sugar, and twice because of the acidity.

· · · · · · · · · · · · · · · · · · · · · · · · · · · · · · · · · · · · · · · · · · · · · ·

**Agave Nectar** —Agave nectar is a high-fructose-containing food masquerading as a health food. It contains as much or more fructose as high fructose corn syrup. Extensive research has shown that is not a raw or unrefined product despite marketing claims to the contrary. Watch out because agave nectar is hiding in many "health food" products such as "health food" bars. There appears to be a disconnection between products marketed as health foods, and what is really healthy to eat.

**Glycerin** —This sweet byproduct was originally from animal fat used in candle making. Now it can come from a variety of sources including biodiesel manufacturing. Although glycerin has many uses, it seems toxic to the body to take internally.

**Malted Grain Sweeteners** —Watch out for malted grains like barley and corn. Either the type of the sugars in the grain, or the plant toxins from the grains, can cause severe tooth decay.

**Brown Rice Syrup** —The sugar in brown rice syrup is recognized by the human body. However, I am very concerned about the presence of grain anti-nutrients, and the enzyme methodology of processing and creating the syrup. The similarity of brown rice syrup to malted barley syrup (which I know promotes cavities significantly) is a cause for serious concern.

**Molasses** —This is a byproduct of beet or cane sugar production. It probably has a similar level of safety to cane sugar in relation to tooth decay, but I am not sure.

**Sugar Isolates** —Maltodextrin, sucrose, dextrose and so forth are isolates of naturally occurring sugars. Avoid these.

**Fake Sweeteners** —These are sucralose, aspartame, and saccharine. A wide body of evidence and concern exists regarding the hazards of artificial sweeteners.

If you want further information about toxic sugars, visit **www.sugarshock-blog.com**

# *Protein for Your Teeth*

Eating protein with each meal balances your blood sugar. Since blood sugar fluctuations over time are a key reason for our body losing minerals, having at least a small amount of protein with every meal will help ensure your body stays biochemically balanced. Protein provides essential body building tools. The higher the quality of protein you eat, as in grass-fed or wild game, the higher quality of protein you will be made up of. Having at least some protein in your diet is absolutely essential to balancing your blood sugar, and to healing tooth cavities.

A nourishing supply of fat, protein and minerals comes from eating animal flesh. Many successful indigenous groups that Dr. Price studied consumed large amounts of animal flesh. Depending on your particular needs and desires, muscle meats can be consumed anywhere on the spectrum from fully cooked to totally raw. Since muscle meats are a common food in our culture, one needs to make sure to balance these with eating enough fat and vegetables. Good quality muscle meat (chicken, beef, fish etc.,) contains phosphorus, amino acids, and other minerals that can build healthy teeth. Vegetarians can obtain protein from eggs and cheese.

· · · · · · · · · · · · · · · · · · · · · · · · · · · · · · · · · · · · · · · · · · · · · · · · · · ·

### Dry Aged Beef
Grass-fed beef can be aged by hanging it in a cold room for several weeks. The beef's natural enzymes tenderize the meat and enhance the flavor. Dry aged beef is a tasty and easy to digest protein.

· · · · · · · · · · · · · · · · · · · · · · · · · · · · · · · · · · · · · · · · · · · · · · · · · · ·

## Protein Assimilation

The flavor of our life is enhanced when we prepare proteins to ensure for maximum taste and digestion. Animal proteins that are not digested properly release toxic by-products into our bodies. When our bodies are healthy—and most people are not in optimal health—the chemical fires of our digestive system neutralize and fully assimilate proteins, and the toxic by-products are easily removed. For the majority of us, cooked animal proteins leave some toxic residues in our bodies.

The cooking methods mentioned here will all significantly increase your ability to safely digest and utilize proteins. Since proteins are body builders, easy to digest proteins in your diet are important to stop tooth decay. Here are some delicious variations to cook proteins that enhance their flavor and digestion.

**Barbecue**—Grill your food on wood coals. This adds a wonderful flavor and juicy texture to your food. Commercially prepared charcoals with chemicals added can make food toxic, but real wood for barbecues leaves your proteins juicy and flavorful.

**Rare** —A well-done steak generally does not taste as good as medium rare or rare. Beef, lamb, and ahi tuna all taste great seared but not fully cooked.

**Stews** —Eating fully cooked proteins with a gelatin-rich broth as stew or as gravy enhances your body's ability to absorb the protein. Cooked protein repels digestive juices in our stomach. But mixing cooked protein with a gelatin-rich broth makes the protein attract digestive juices and digest well.

**Raw** —Our culture's many cuisines are full of raw protein foods; we just do not usually notice. Body builders consume raw eggs in smoothies. Other common raw foods are: steak tartare, sushi and sashimi, cheese, and oysters. I usually have no problems eating certain types of animal foods raw. Other people prefer to freeze or marinate animal proteins before they consume them raw to destroy possible pathogens. Raw protein can be very easy to digest because it absorbs water.

**Chemical "Cooking"** —Surprisingly we have fermented raw meats available in our culture. Salami, cold smoked salmon, and corned beef are a few examples. Ceviche is an example where acid from lemon or lime cooks the food (raw fish) while it marinates. These types of no-heat cooking methods make protein easy to digest and taste good.

## Protein Balance

The different ways to cook and prepare proteins are designed to increase your assimilation of protein and hopefully help heal any intestinal damage or poor digestion. Eating a high protein diet does not work for many people because we need to eat adequate amounts of fat with our proteins. So do not be shy about enjoying fat with your protein. Proteins go well in combination with vegetables or grains.

Many people have slightly damaged intestinal walls where partially digested protein can permeate directly into the bloodstream.[125] If you have this condition, you generally will not feel very well after eating a lot of protein. In the worst case your joints could swell in an autoimmune reaction to the proteins in your bloodstream. Eating small amounts of proteins with larger amounts of cooked vegetables helps people with problems assimilating protein. Dentist Melvin Page estimated that we should eat a minimum of 1/15th of our body weight in protein per day. To get your minimum or average protein intake, take your desired body weight and divide it by 15. For example, someone who weighs 150 pounds should eat at least 10 ounces of protein spread throughout the day. Dr. Page thought that more small meals with protein spread throughout the day would help control and balance your blood sugar. You can eat more protein than this, but for most people less than this amount is not advisable.

# Low Quality Proteins

Factory-farmed meats and eggs promote a profit-driven system of disease in which animals are misused and mistreated. The cesspools from these factory farms pollute the air and the environment including water supplies. Factory-farmed animals many times are barely allowed to move, are loaded with drugs and chemicals to keep them alive, and are not fed their natural diet. It is unwise to eat the unhealthy meat from these animals. Choose fresh grass-fed meats whenever possible.

Conventional packaged lunch meats contain many harmful food additives. Avoid those. Organic packaged meats like salami, bacon, hotdogs, sausages and so forth can be health-promoting but it really depends on how they are processed and what ingredients are added. Use those foods with caution to ensure they are not negatively affecting your health.

## *Protein Powders*

I know of some case studies in which people got tooth decay from consuming protein powder. The significant processing of most protein powders renders the protein hazardous. Some high-quality protein powders made from high-quality animal foods <u>may</u> be of benefit to people, but this is not known for certain. What is the point of consuming protein powder when you can have real, healthy protein? For example: If whey protein is healthy, then simply drink whey every day. That way you get safe protein and probiotics as an added bonus. If you feel that you need more protein in your diet then have real and natural proteins like eggs, fish, or beef. Soy protein blocks iron absorption even when all the phytic acid has been removed;[126] this is an example of one of the many hazards of protein powders.

## *Phosphorus*

Phosphorus is perhaps even more important to tooth remineralization than calcium. Phosphorous is in most foods. However it is highly concentrated in dairy products like milk and cheese, in the organs of land and sea animals, in muscle meats and proteins including eggs, and in grains, nuts and beans. One has to be careful in using grains and beans for phosphorous sources because some grains, like white rice, do not contain much phosphorous. Meanwhile other whole grains contain phosphorous in a form that is not absorbable. Vegetables do not contain much phosphorous. Three and a half ounces of a hard cheese provides 0.6 grams of phosphorus; the same amount of beef, chicken or fish contains about 0.25 grams. Four cups of raw milk provide 0.9 grams of phosphorus. Organ meats are generally much richer in phosphorous than muscle meats. Dr. Price's nutritional recommendation for phosphorus is 2.0 grams per day. This recommendation is double the US National Academy of Sciences dietary reference intake.

**Eggs**
4 eggs contain 0.5 grams of phosphorous. Eggs from pastured chickens, ducks or other animals are rich in tooth-decay-fighting vitamins and minerals.

## Fermented Foods & Enzymes

Enzymes act as catalysts in most of the biochemical processes in our bodies. When we cook our food completely at temperatures above 150°F, its enzyme content is destroyed. When you eat a cooked meal, it is vital to include and consume both raw and/or fermented foods with the cooked food. Enzymes help us digest our foods. One way to get these enzymes is through the use of fermented foods. Fermented drinks include rejuvelac, kefir, and beet kvass. Fermented foods include fermented radish, cabbage (sauerkraut), pickles, fermented sweet potatoes and yogurt. Fermented vegetables are a great way to consume your vegetables. Recipes for fermented foods can be found in *Nourishing Traditions* by Sally Fallon. Taking enzyme supplements or high quality probiotics is another method to help your body assimilate food and achieve balance.

**Fermented or Uncooked Food**
Have something raw or fermented with every meal that otherwise is of exclusively cooked food.

## Vegetables for Minerals

We are told to cook our meat, chicken or fish completely to avoid harmful bacteria. Meanwhile even many health-oriented people think we should have our vegetables raw to preserve nutrients and enzymes. But uncooked vegetables contain a host of plant toxins including enzyme inhibitors, oxalates, saponins, and lectins. Besides a few exceptions such as lettuce or cucumber, raw vegetables are difficult to digest. Only people with strong digestive powers can do well eating lots of uncooked vegetables. For the rest of us, we need heat or fermentation to break down the vegetable cellulose. Unless you have very strong digestive fires, eating a great deal of raw vegetables is not healthy because of the plant toxins. Vegetables should be prepared such that they should be easy to digest and assimilate, as well as taste good.

If you visit a farm you can watch goats or cows madly salivate over grass. I have noticed that reaction does not occur with humans. That is because we are not made to eat too many uncooked raw fibrous vegetables. Raw vegetables can irritate the intestinal lining especially if the lining is already inflamed. Cooked vegetables and fruits have their cellulose broken down so they are easier for us to digest. I recommend usually eating cooked vegetables or fruit with some type of fat like butter or cream. To me, a soft cooked piece of broccoli with some butter or cheese is much easier to digest than a piece of raw crunchy broccoli. When vegetables are juiced, the cellulose is removed and the nutrients are free to be assimilated. However too much vegetable juice may expose you to unnecessary plant toxins and even excess sugars, depending upon which vegetables you are juicing.

Dark, leafy-green vegetables need to be eaten cooked, as the nutrients are released through cooking. The bottom line is to prepare your vegetables in a way that tastes good to you. Do not force yourself to eat raw vegetables to try to be healthy.

## Are Grains the Hidden Reason for many Modern Diseases including Tooth Cavities?

9,000 years ago around 7,000 BC wheat and barley were first cultivated. Corn and rice followed 2,500 years later in 4,500 BC. According to human fossil records, prior to this time period, tooth decay was virtually unknown. Teeth recovered from Pakistan dating to around 5,500 BC show signs of being drilled, presumably because of cavities. For the last 5,000 years the average rate of tooth decay has been climbing. The rise in the rate of tooth decay has also been seen in Native Americans who switched from a hunter gatherer lifestyle to a more heavily corn-based diet.[127] The cultivation of grains has fostered the evolution of civilization, allowing city centers to emerge in which large groups of people live together such as in ancient Egypt. Grains also made it possible to raise large armies as it resolved the logistical problem of feeding thousands of soldiers.

In Weston Price's field studies, a diet centered on white flour, refined sugar and vegetable fats was devastating to the health, teeth and gums of native peoples worldwide. From this evidence even Dr. Price himself concluded that consuming grain products in their whole form would resolve a part of the problem of tooth decay. The natural health community, and now even the US Government and food manufacturing giants, have embraced and promoted the view that whole grains are better for our health.

Beyond the fossil evidence connecting grains to tooth cavities is over one hundred years of scientific research that connects whole grains with a variety of diseases. This evidence is further consistently confirmed by the nearly daily e-mails I receive from stressed-out healthy eaters wondering why their previously cavity-free children now have tooth decay. There is one clear response that over and over again proves to be correct: whole grains.

Considering modern humans (*Homo sapiens*) are about 200,000 years old, large amounts of grains constitute a very recent addition to the modern diet. Our bodies are not designed to eat grains in their raw form so grains require us to use our intelligence to predigest the grains through the process of fermentation and then cooking. In the absence of careful grain preparation including fermentation, a host of diseases appear.

The famous professor and doctor Edward Mellanby wrote that "oatmeal and grain embryo interfere most strongly" with the building of healthy teeth. He called the effect of the germ of grains on teeth "baneful." He also found that a diet high in grain germ or embryo led to nervous system problems in his dogs such as leg weakness and uncoordinated movements. Dr. Mellanby concluded that most cereals contain a toxic substance that can affect the nervous system.[128] He pointed out the connection of grains and legumes to pellagra, a niacin deficiency, lathyrism, which is immobility caused by bean toxins in the lathyrus family such as a certain type of sweet pea, and pernicious anemia which is related to a vitamin $B_{12}$ deficiency. Each one of these diseases is most effectively treated with animal liver. And each one of these diseases can be produced in laboratory conditions by feeding whole grains.

## The Anti-Scorbutic Vitamin and Your Teeth and Gums

Scurvy was made famous as a common disease among sailors. It occurred after long sea voyages when sailors had to subsist on dried foods including dried grain products such as hard tack. The symptoms of scurvy include soft and spongy gums which eventually lead to tooth loss, slow wound healing, poor bone formation, severe weakness, nausea and eventually death. Gum disease is a major factor in tooth loss as we age. We learned from dentist W.D. Miller that healthy gums protect teeth from tooth decay. Since tooth loss from gum disease is a symptom of scurvy, it is feasible that what causes and cures scurvy might cause and cure gum problems as well.

Researchers were excited to discover an animal model with which to practice scurvy experiments. Guinea pigs fed a high grain diet developed a condition that appears to be exactly the same as scurvy in humans. [129] To cause scurvy, guinea pigs were fed mostly bran and oats. Another scurvy-producing diet consisted of whole grains like oats, barley, maize, and soy bean flour. An exclusive oatmeal diet would kill a guinea pig in 24 days from scurvy. This very same scurvy-inducing diet produced severe tooth and gum problems in guinea pigs as well.

That whole grains are the cause of scurvy sheds light on the severity of plant toxins found naturally in grains. Guinea pigs fed germinated oats and barley did not contract scurvy.[130] This reveals that the sprouting process may disable anti-nutrients that cause scurvy. Research on scurvy eventually led to the discovery of the anti-scorbutic (anti-scurvy) vitamin which we know as vitamin C. **Reintroducing vitamin C in the diet of guinea pigs with raw cabbage (sauerkraut would work for humans) or orange juice resolves the disease.**

Some scurvy researchers suspected that the lack of vitamin C was not the essential cause of scurvy. Rather they believed that vitamin C protected against some injurious factor in the diet. Since a scurvy-inducing diet largely consisted of whole grains, perhaps the injurious factor is something in the grains. Today we know that grains contain numerous plant toxins and anti-nutrients including lectins and phytic acid.

Phytic acid is the principal storage form of phosphorus in many plant tissues, especially the bran portion of grains and other seeds. It is found in significant amounts in grains, nuts, beans, seeds, and some tubers. Phytic acid contains the mineral phosphorus tightly bound in a snowflake-like molecule. In humans and animals with one stomach, the phosphorus is not readily bioavailable. In addition to blocking phosphorus availability, the "arms" of the phytic acid molecule readily bind with other minerals, such as calcium, magnesium, iron and zinc, making them unavailable as well. Yet the negative effects of phytic acid can be significantly reduced with vitamin C. Adding vitamin C to the diet can significantly counteract phytic acid's iron absorption blocking effect.[131] This leaves us with compelling evidence that the symptoms of scurvy like soft and spongy gums leading to tooth loss are the result of a lack of vitamin C, and too many grains, or other phytic acid-rich foods. Perhaps vitamin C's remarkable ability to heal and prevent scurvy is because of its ability to aid in iron absorption which was disturbed by too many improperly prepared grains rich in phytic acid.

Giving rats and dogs a scurvy-producing diet did not lead to scurvy, it led to another disease, rickets. Rickets is a disease that is known for producing severely bowed legs in children. Other rickets symptoms include muscle weakness, bone pain or tenderness, skeletal problems and tooth decay. To produce rickets in the laboratory, dogs were fed oatmeal. Professor Edward Mellanby describes his findings of decades of research:

> [M]ore severe rickets developed when the diet consisted mainly of oatmeal, maize or whole wheat flour than when these substances were replaced by equal amounts of either white flour or rice, in spite of the fact that the former cereals contained more calcium and phosphorus than the latter.[132]

The most severe rickets-producing diet was a mostly whole grain diet which included whole wheat, whole corn, and wheat gluten.[133] Rickets has been identified as a disease of calcium, phosphorous and vitamin D metabolism.[134] In one study, hospital cases of rickets fell greatly in June.[135] As previously mentioned,

Activator X-rich butter was shown to prevent rickets. This is because Activator X would appear in high quantities in June grass-fed butter. Germination of oats itself did not reduce the rickets- producing effect of whole oats. But germination together with fermentation of whole grains greatly reduced the severity of rickets.[136] On the rickets-producing diet, teeth become abnormal. There is a known impairment of the ability for teeth to mineralize that is associated with rickets. In rare cases of rickets, some children's teeth do not erupt. Rickets is cured or prevented by having adequate fat-soluble vitamin D in the diet. This is because vitamin D increases the utilization of phosphorous and calcium in diets with phytic acid, and without phytic acid.

Scurvy and rickets are both produced in laboratory experiments in different animals using a diet consisting largely of whole grains. The connection between scurvy and rickets is not a random coincidence; it has also been observed in humans. Dr. Thomas Barlow of England carefully studied rickets cases in children, and published a report in 1883 suggesting that scurvy and rickets are closely related.[137] Infantile scurvy is also known as Barlow's Disease. Both scurvy and rickets are connected to serious problems with teeth and/or gums. It seems both possible and reasonable that whole grains can cause scurvy in the absence of vitamin C, and rickets in the absence of vitamin D.

Scurvy still occurs in modern times, and the cause is still the same. In one previously healthy individual, strictly following a macrobiotic diet nearly caused death from scurvy within one year. Her diet consisted mostly of whole brown rice and other freshly ground whole grains.[138]

## The Effect of Oats on Children's Teeth

It is not just in animal experiments that teeth disintegrate from consumption of whole grains. Dr. May Mellanby published several articles in the prestigious *British Medical Journal* about food and tooth decay from 1924 –1932. Multiple investigations were done to show the effect of oatmeal and fat-soluble vitamins on children's teeth. The children studied already had numerous cavities. A grain-free diet high in fat-soluble vitamins A and D from cod liver oil produced the best results, with essentially no new cavities forming. These grain-free children also showed signs of their decayed teeth remineralizing. The tooth-healing diet included milk, meat, eggs, butter, potatoes and cod liver oil. [139]

By accident medical doctor J.D. Boyd healed diabetic children's decayed teeth by designing a grain-free diet. The diet meant to control diabetes not only stopped cavities it turned soft tooth enamel hard and glossy. These findings were published in 1928 in the *Journal of the American Medical Association*. Dr. Boyd's diet consisted of milk, cream, butter, eggs, meat, cod liver oil, vegetables and fruit. Please note that both Dr. Mellanby's and Dr. Boyd's tooth-remineralizing diet came from a time when milk, butter and cream were raw, farm-fresh and grass-fed.

Meanwhile in two other feeding experiments by Dr. Mellanby a low fat-soluble vitamin A and D diet with the addition of ½ to 1 cup of oatmeal per day produced an average of six new cavities per child during the trial period. Their preexisting cavities did not heal in any way. A diet with less oatmeal and some fat-soluble vitamins produced an average of four and a half new cavities per child, with a few of the preexisting cavities healing during the experiment.[140] The take-home message from these experiments is that oatmeal has a devastating effect on teeth, and that the maximum amount of bone growth and tooth remineralization in these studies occurred with grain-free diets.

Both Edward and May Mellanby's decades of research show that oatmeal interferes more than any other grain studied with tooth mineralization. Intermediate interference of tooth mineralization occurs from corn, rye, barley and rice. Wheat germ, corn germ and other grain germs have a "baneful" effect on teeth. **White flour interferes the least** with tooth mineralization.[141] That white flour does not interfere as much with tooth mineralization corresponds with Weston Price's feeding experiments discussed in chapter two in which cavity-ridden school children consumed two meals per day consisting of white flour, and one excellent meal per day with nutrient-dense foods. Even while consuming the white flour the children all became immune to tooth cavities. In human nutrient absorption experiments, in diets with mostly whole wheat flour (8% of grain solids removed) calcium, magnesium, phosphorus and potassium were less completely absorbed than a more refined flour (with 21% of grain solids removed).[142] If white flour interfered the least with tooth remineralization you might wonder why native people on a white flour diet succumbed to tooth decay. The answer lies in the fact that white flour in general either replaced more nutrient-dense foods or that in a context of a low mineral, high sugar diet, white flour was disastrous for teeth. Had white flour been consumed with cod's heads and cod's liver, or raw milk cheese the results would be different. (Note: I do not advocate white flour consumption.) Rather white flour was consumed generally with sugar in the form of pastries, or with jam and jelly on toast.

The long chain of beliefs that have led to the modern conclusion that whole grains are healthy to eat comes without looking at the complete body of evidence. The problems seen with whole grains primarily lie in the toxic properties Dr. Mellanby identified residing in the bran and the germ. Grain toxicity is then exponentially magnified by the absence of vitamins C and D in our diet which protect against grain toxins. Conversely, overly processed and mishandled grains, particularly white flour, have their own host of health consequences. The answer to healthy grain consumption lies in the middle ground of not overly processed, and not minimally processed.

Experiments with sprouted grains showed that oats and corn that are first sprouted and then soured at room temperature for two days (thus eliminating large amounts of anti-nutrients) lost their ability to produce rickets.[143] While germinated and then soured grains do not produce rickets, they do not create optimal bone growth unless there is sufficient vitamin D in the diet.[144]

# Problems with Unfermented Grains

Phytic acid has a strong inhibitory effect on mineral absorption in adults, particularly on the absorption of iron.[145] Even a small amount of phytic acid in one's diet can lead to a significant reduction in iron absorption. While grains, particularly whole grains, are rich in phosphorous, up to 80% of this phosphorous is bound up as phytate, which is not absorbable by the body.[146] Phytic acid inhibits enzymes that we need to digest our food, including pepsin,[147] which is needed for the breakdown of proteins in the stomach, and amylase,[148] which is required for the breakdown of starch into sugar. Trypsin, needed for protein digestion in the small intestine, is also inhibited by phytic acid.[149] The concentration of and types of enzyme inhibitors varies considerably between different types of grains.[150] Grains also contain tannins which can depress growth, decrease iron absorption, and damage the mucosal lining of the gastrointestinal tract. In addition to tannins, saponins in grains may inhibit growth.[151]

Since phosphorous is the crucial mineral to tooth remineralization we want to then eliminate the bound phosphorous as phytic acid as much as possible from our diet. When it cannot be eliminated, then complementary vitamins and minerals from foods will need to be used: in particular calcium, vitamin C and vitamin D to block phytic acid's effects.

## *LSD in Whole Grains?*

Most, if not all, grains seem to contain nerve toxins, however in different concentrations. Oats and wheat germ seem to contain the highest concentration of these toxins, and white flour much less. Dr. Mellanby referred to this unknown toxin as a toxamin, a toxic substance that is blocked by the presence of vitamins in the diet, particularly fat-soluble vitamins A and D.[152]

The nervous system toxins in many or all beans and grains may explain their insidious effects on teeth. Dr. Mellanby thought the toxin in grains is the same toxin that causes ergot poisoning when grains like rye are infected with a fungus.[153] The interesting note about ergot poisoning is that it can be transferred from the mother to child through breastmilk. It first affects the digestive system, and then the nervous system. In severe cases it also causes seizures and LSD-like effects.

Through examining the diets of people with severe tooth decay I find two patterns. One is an extreme excess of sugar consumption, either from natural sources or from refined fructose. The other is a moderate consumption of whole grains, **regardless of whether the grains are soured or not**. The effect of the grain toxin on teeth appears very similar to someone ingesting large quantities of synthetic fructose syrup.

Since lectins are a sugar-binding protein, it seems that the toxic substance in grains could be lectins or similar grain sugars. Lectins are also found in high amounts in beans. Many types of lectins are easily neutralized by cooking, fermenting, or digestion. Grain's baneful effect on teeth may be a combination of many grain toxins like phytic acid and lectins together. Some lectins cannot be broken down by fermentation or digestion and become poison to our bodies; others are not harmful to humans at all. Agglutinin is a lectin in wheat germ that passes through digestion and into the body and produces intestinal inflammation.

Certain lectins are very poisonous. Ricin, the lectin in castor beans, is lethal to humans in even small doses. It destroys cells by affecting their ability to utilize proteins. Lectins in general can bind to the villi and cells in the small intestine resulting in a diminished capacity for digestion and absorption.[154] In particular lectins can interfere with hormone and growth factor signaling which may explain why they could promote severe cavities or other growth problems. A demonstration of lectins' connection with tooth decay can be shown in a saliva test for lectins that indicates one's susceptibility to tooth decay.[155]

# The Effects of Soaking and Sprouting on Phytic Acid

Scientific studies give us insights into the means to remove phytic acid from grains. Sprouting grains is a wonderful step in the fermentation process. But it does not remove that much phytic acid. Typically sprouting will remove somewhere between 20-30% of phytic acid after two or three days for beans, seeds, and grains[156] under laboratory conditions at a constant 77 degrees Fahrenheit.[157] Sprouting was more effective in rye, rice, millet and mung beans, removing about 50% of phytic acid, and not effective at all with oats. Soaking by itself for 16 hours at a constant 77 degrees typically removed 5-10% of the grain and bean phytic acid content. Soaking increased or did not reduce the phytic acid content of quinoa, sorghum, corn, oats, amaranth, wheat, mung beans and some seeds.[158] These statistics do not illustrate the entire picture. Even though soaking quinoa actually increased phytic acid contents, soaking and then cooking quinoa reduces its phytic acid levels by more than 61%.[159] The same holds true for beans. Soaking and then cooking removes about 50% of phytic acid. With lentils this same procedure removes 76% of phytic acid.[160] Roasting wheat, barley or green gram reduces phytic acid by about 40%.[161] A very interesting report shows the value of grain and bean storage in relation to plant toxins. In humid and warm storage conditions beans lost 65% of their phytic acid content.[162]

# Grain Bran and Fiber

**Grain bran is high in insoluble fiber that your body cannot digest**. This explains the usual indigenous practice to remove grain bran through sifting or other methods. While bran is a fine food for mice, and has been used as an animal feed, these plastic-like substances are not good for humans. Even bran used as fertilizer needs to be fermented to release its vitamins. Many indigenous cultures process their food to make it soft, tasty, and easy to digest. When I was younger I believed the premise that bran was healthy because it had lots of nutrients. So I would force myself to eat bran muffins. Even with the large amount of unhealthy sugar, the bran muffins tasted terrible. I was not listening to what my body wanted when eating the bran. My body did not want to eat bran; it wanted to spit it out. The benefits of fiber from bran are unproven. The large bulky material may irritate your digestive tract. Bran-enriched food, especially bran that is not thoroughly fermented, will have extremely high amounts of demineralizing phytic acid. Focus on foods that taste good and are easy to digest and absorb rather than foods that the television or government says are good but that your body feels repelled by.

# Indigenous People's Fermentation of Grain

It is difficult to hand tailor the available information on grain and legume toxicity and transform it into guidelines for making all grains safe to eat. Each type of grain has a substantially individual botanical structure. Further, each grain species has regional differences; for example, there are more than 50,000 known varieties of wheat.[163] The concentration of grain toxins may vary widely based on the particular grain and its regional variety.

To make grain, nut, legume, and seed consumption healthy we need to remove as much phytic acid and other grain toxins as possible. Because each grain, nut, bean or seed is its own entity, each requires different types of attention to make it safe to eat. How safe grains are for you to eat varies greatly based on your genetic lineage, how old you are (kids are far more susceptible to wrongly prepared grains), how efficient your digestion is, how many grains, nuts, seeds and beans you consume, and what other foods you eat.

Indigenous people went through extreme lengths to process their grains to make them healthy to eat. In our modern culture we do not go to these same lengths, and suffer as a result. The lesson I have learned from the proper preparation of grains and beans is that there are no shortcuts. One wrong move with them, and your teeth might be crumbling apart. Food fermentation preserves food, enriches the vitamin and amino acid content, removes plant toxins, and decreases the cooking time. Grains that are prepared for alcoholic beverages are at first sprouted.

## *Rye, Wheat, Spelt, Kamut, and Barley*

Indigenous cultures know how to prepare grains and beans properly to ensure optimal health. In the Loetschental Valley in Dr. Price's time the natives did not have doctors or dentists because they did not need them. They also consumed large amounts of sourdough rye bread. A careful analysis of the Swiss diet nutrient chart earlier in this book shows that the high alpine rye bread only provides a little bit more than 0.1 grams of phosphorous in the daily diet than white bread. This is not the huge difference in nutrients that whole grains are supposed to have over white flour. The explanation for this is that the people of the Swiss Alps did not use the whole rye grain.

As in many cultures across the world, the Swiss natives started with a whole rye kernel. But after grinding it slowly on a stone wheel, they sifted the rye and removed approximately ¼ of the flour mixture by weight of all impurities.[164] Bran and germ consist of approximately 15-20% of the entire kernel. To be clear, if they started with one cup of flour, after sifting they would have ¾ of a cup of flour remaining. This rye bread still probably contained trace amounts of bran and germ vitamins. Even without knowing the science of phytic acid and lectins, they removed the phytic acid through fermentation, and removed toxic lectins in the germ and bran of the rye grain by sifting out the germ and the bran completely. It is likely then that the safe consumption of our most common grains similar to rye, like wheat, kamut, spelt, and barley involve a substantial or complete removal of the bran and the germ. The high Alpine natives produced a sourdough rye bread in large batches, which included a four-and-a-half-hour hand mixing time.[165] While the people in the Loetschental Valley baked their bread once per month, a more ancient recipe was based upon only one single communal bread baking per year. That means for the rest of the year the bread aged while it was hung on walls. There is evidence that aging grains under certain conditions removes phytic acid and it may also further degrade other grain toxins.

When considering healthy grain consumption we often overlook the importance of the other foods eaten with the grains. How healthy a grain is to eat for the health of your teeth depends on how much phytic acid and other toxins the grain has as well as how much or how little calcium is in your diet. The Swiss natives who enjoyed near total immunity to tooth decay understood this principle and combined their rye bread consumption with cheese and milk in the same meal. This food combining of calcium-rich cheese and milk, and vitamin C-rich dairy products protected them against any residual grain toxins left in their bread not destroyed by milling, fermentation, sifting, baking and aging. The secret to the healthy Loetschental Valley people is their preparation methods which produced grains low in toxins, as well as their consumption of grains in combination with dairy products which were high in calcium, phosphorous, and fat-soluble vitamins.

Wheat and dairy products eaten together is not just seen in the high Alpine villages. In Africa a traditional dish made from wheat known as kishk involves a laborious process to make the wheat safe to eat. First the wheat is boiled, dried, and then ground. The bran is completely removed as in the case of the Loetschental rye preparation. Milk is soured in a separate vessel, and then milk and bran-free wheat are soured together for 24–48 hours, and finally dried for storage.

Ancient beer recipes do use the bran and germ of grains. Ancient beer is a fermentation method that extracts the good vitamins from the bran and the germ without exposing the beer drinker to the grain toxins. Unfortunately modern commercially brewed beers can cause cavities.

## Healthy Oats

The Gaelics of the Outer Hebrides regularly consumed large amounts of oats, but they did not suffer from scurvy, rickets, or tooth decay. In contrast, rickets was very common in more modern parts of Scotland where oats were also consumed. The difference between the two oat-eating groups was the fat-soluble content of their diets, and how the oats were prepared. Oats were stored outdoors after harvesting and the oats partially germinated for days or even weeks in the rain and sun.[166] The outer husk was collected and fermented for a week or longer. This could have been used to produce an enzyme-rich starter for souring oats. Oats may have been fermented anywhere from 12–24 hours and as long as a week. I am unclear if the oats were consumed whole, or if the bran was removed. I am further unclear on all the details on how oats were prepared. Modern oatmeal flakes typically have the bran removed. The diet of the Outer Hebrides was extremely rich in fat-soluble vitamins A and D from cod's head stuffed with cod livers which would protect against phytic acid. Their diet was also very rich in minerals from consumption of shellfish which could replenish potentially lost or blocked minerals if there was any phytic acid left in the oats. The combination of soil tending, careful oat preparation, and a mineral- and fat-soluble rich diet allowed oats to be a healthy staple for the isolated Gaelic populations.

Unlike the careful harvesting and storage of oats by isolated cultures, even organic whole oats you buy in the store are heat treated and they are not left in the fields to germinate and dry. Oats are heat treated because the high fat content of this grain can easily suffer rancidity during storage. The heat treated oats lose their entire phytase enzyme content however, so soaking or souring oatmeal will not destroy any phytic acid prior to cooking. There is a surprising percentage of people I have talked to who have cavities or whose children have cavities who are heavy oat eaters. This confirms the results of the Mellanby's years of human and animal trials. In the rickets experiments, oats that are first sprouted and then soured for two days lost their ability to produce rickets.

The problem with preparing truly healthy-to-eat oats is that you need to special order oats that are still alive in order to sprout them. I am uncertain if you can make heat treated oats safe for the health of your teeth. My suggestion would be to sprout oats for two days and then to dry them and remove the oat bran through grinding and sifting or flaking. Then you would need to sour oats at a warm temperature with a starter for 24 hours before consuming. The consequences of oats that are not expertly prepared for our teeth are a documented cause for concern.

## Healthy Rice

In rice-eating countries across the globe, rice is rarely consumed in its brown form, with the whole bran. In a quest to find the most ancient and traditional preparation methods, I found several accounts of partially polished rice. Rice is traditionally stored in its husk, and then fresh pounded before cooking. How much bran is removed in traditional brown rice preparation seems to be dependent on the breed of rice, and the other foods available in the diet. Ancient rice preparation included low tech milling, such as tumbling the rice with stones which removes a significant portion of bran and germ from the rice.[167] But some portion of the bran and germ remain. That exact amount of bran to be removed will depend on how long the rice is fermented, and the specific type of rice used. A good guess would be 50% of bran should be removed from rice. Milled rice has usually a little bit of germ, polished rice no germ.

Rancid rice has a bitter aftertaste. In several nutrient absorption studies brown rice consumption did not lead to more nutrient absorption compared to rice with the bran removed. In one specific study, brown rice was compared with milled rice (rice without most of the bran and germ, but not polished totally white). There was no difference in nutrient absorption even though the brown rice actually contained more nutrients.[168] This apparent contradiction would be explained by the phytic acid and other anti-nutrients in the rice. One study showed that the anti-iron phytate levels in rice were disabled by the vitamin C in collard greens.[169] Because rice goes rancid rapidly or because insects and rodents eat it quickly, in rice-eating cultures rice is stored in the husk, or stored as white rice. In most of the rice-eating populations across the world it is very difficult to find brown rice.

In a rice-based diet rice toxins are neutralized by sour fruit and vegetables high in vitamin C, land or sea organ meats rich in fat-soluble vitamins, and sometimes via the fermentation of rice or beans. Completely bran- and germ-free rice, known as white rice, can cause a vitamin B–1 (thiamine) deficiency in a diet very high in or exclusively of white rice. The condition is known as beriberi. Beriberi rarely occurred in people eating partially milled rice which retained a small portion of the bran. I know of people in rice-eating cultures with beautiful white, cavity-free teeth who grew up on white rice.

Brem is a special rice-cake bread from Indonesia. It goes through a truly heroic fermentation process in which the rice is fermented for 5–6 days, and then it is sun dried for an additional 5–7 days. Millet and rice are also traditionally fermented with fish, pork or shrimp for several weeks to produce fermented condiments. The healthiest rice I have eaten is a partially milled rice (it has streaks of bran on it) that has been soaked with the brown rice starter as described in chapter six.

## Healthy Corn

Even more than rice, the healthy preparation of corn as a grain is largely dependent upon the variety of the corn being used. This leads to a wide variety of traditional corn preparation methods which range from simple roasting to fermenting for two weeks.

Corn is universally nixtamalized when prepared for consumption as flour. This is a process of soaking corn in an alkaline solution to release niacin (vitamin $B_3$) and then hulling. Modern corn tortillas, chips, and corn meals have either no corn bran or germ, or have very little corn bran or germ. They also are nixtamalized. Typical corn products with the bran and germ removed would be lower in phytic acid and lower in toxic properties than whole grain corn. I cannot clearly advise on how much of these corn products is safe to eat in relation to dental health. They seem comparable to unfermented unbleached wheat flour. If a food has the entire corn kernel in it, and it has not gone through a thorough fermentation process it probably is very high in anti-nutrients like phytic acid and lectins. I am certain that food products containing the entire corn kernel, either as it is, or as sprouted corn should be avoided. Another issue of concern with corn is genetically modified corn. Because of cross pollination, even many not genetically modified corns may have some genetic alteration. Animals typically will not eat genetically modified (GM) corn unless they are forced to do so. Those that have eaten it have had reproductive problems among other problems.

Ogi, a traditional fermented cereal from West Africa illustrates the efforts needed to make corn, sorghum or millet safe to eat for children. To begin, the grains are already sun dried after harvesting and stored in their hulls. The corn is then soaked for 1–3 days. The corn bran, corn hulls, and corn germ are completely removed. The mixture is then fermented for 2–3 days, cooked and then dried for storage.[170]

Pozol is a fermented corn dish from South America. The corn is cooked with calcium hydroxide to release niacin. The hull, or pericarp, of the corn is removed. Pozol is fermented for 1–14 days.

Not every single indigenous grain recipe removes the bran of the grain or even ferments the grain. Injera is an Ethiopian bread traditionally made from teff. The recipe I have for injera uses from whole grain sorghum. The sorghum is fermented with an enzyme-rich starter for 48 hours. Chapati is a flat bread from India made with whole wheat and it is not leavened. In both of these cases it appears the cultures took a recipe that was fine with one grain, such as teff in Ethiopia and rice in India, and then used that same recipe with another more recently introduced grain. Over the past several hundred years new levels of trading, immigration and adoption of customs from other cultures have created whole grain recipes that appear superficially to be traditional, but are in fact adopted and do not effectively remove grain toxins.

Sometimes it requires digging deep to find truly ancient and holistic grain recipes. There are so many examples of time-consuming and energy-intensive grain processing methods. If it was possible for cultures using these intensive methods of grain preparation to be healthy with less work, or to retain a higher yield by keeping the bran and the germ, I am certain they would have done so. I therefore believe these slow fermented and time-consuming ways of preparing grains, typically with the bran and germ removed, are the ones which will produce the greatest degree of health.

## Characteristics of Indigenous People's Grain Preparation

- Biodynamic soil practices.

- Careful grain harvesting, including slow drying in the sun.

- Aging of grains.

- Storing grains carefully, many times with the outer hull to preserve freshness.

- Grinding grains fresh before preparation.

- Combining grains with other foods.

- Generally removing the bran and/or germ from the grain.

- Use of starters in low-phytase grains.

## Phytic Acid Content of Popular Foods

**Avoid Commercially Made Whole Grain Products**—Yeasted breads have 40-80% of their phytic acid intact in their finished product.[171] If a yeasted bread is made with unbleached white flour, however, it will not have much phytic acid. I have cited numerous examples of the problems with grain bran and germ, and demonstrated that these problems are eliminated by removing the grain bran and germ. There is a big price to pay for not removing most of the bran and germ in the grains in the grass family including wheat, rye, spelt, kamut, and barley. I have heard of several cases now of whole wheat sourdough with spelt causing severe tooth decay. This is because fermentation, while good at removing phytic acid, does not neutralize all the grain toxins like lectins in certain types and varieties of grains. This leads me to the conclusion that it is best to avoid commercially prepared breads, crackers, health food bars, pastas, cereals and anything else in the store that contains whole grains. No exceptions. Since quinoa and buckwheat are pseudo cereals and not exactly grains, there is some chance that they can be consumed whole provided you remove the phytic acid. But I do not know this for certain. Without knowing what the exact toxin is in the grains causing severe cavities, and without specifically testing each particular store-bought food, I cannot say that any whole grain foods from the store will keep your teeth safe from tooth decay.

**Avoid sprouted grain breads** —Another deadly food for teeth is commercially made sprouted grain products from whole grains. The whole grain plant toxins are not sufficiently neutralized by sprouting and these foods can cause severe tooth decay.

**Avoid most gluten-free grain products**—Many gluten-free products are made with brown rice. Brown rice will be very high in phytic acid and these products should be avoided. Gluten-free grain products made from white rice, on the other hand, will not have much phytic acid or grain toxins.

**Avoid breakfast cereals**—These now have bran or whole grains added to them for the advertised fiber and supposed health features of bran. Cereals with whole grains will be very high in phytic acid and likely high in other grain toxins.

**Avoid health food bars** —Many contain whole grains that are not properly soured and are very high in grain toxins. They also contain lots of sugar.

**Limit popcorn**—Popcorn has some phytic acid. Definitely avoid it if you have tooth decay. Moderate amounts of popcorn are safe to eat for people who are otherwise healthy.

# Safe Grains Guidelines

## *Low Phytic Acid, and Low Lectin Grains*

Here are introductory guidelines that are easy to follow which reduce or eliminate the possibility that grains will harm your teeth. You want your grains to be as free from plant toxins as possible. These guidelines are for grains that are safe for the health of your teeth and that are easy to obtain. Many of the grain products available today are compromise foods. I therefore do not recommend them as part of an ideal diet but they should be adequate. For the reader who wants excellent improvement in dental health without spending hours in the kitchen fussing about grains, this part is for you.

Semolina is the name for the part of the wheat left over after removing the bran and the germ. It is used to make pasta and couscous. It is unclear how healthy these unfermented processed grains are to eat, but they will be low in phytic acid if they are not made from whole grains. Traditionally couscous and pasta would be made from semolina or other bran-free grains that are soured or fermented in some way. These options are not available commercially as far as I know.

Any type of bread made with unbleached white flour will be low in phytic acid. Fermented sourdough bread is the ideal way to consume unbleached flour. Sourdough bread with unbleached flour that is sour in taste is the best grain product available in the western world. Not all sourdoughs are created equally. The bread should be soured at least 16 hours and be sour in taste. Some artisan bakers even freshly grind the whole wheat or rye, and remove the bran and germ to make an excellent soured loaf.

White rice does not have much phytic acid. It appears that white jasmine and white basmati rice in health food stores retain a tiny portion of the rice germ because of their brownish color. White rice does not seem to have negative health effects on people like white flour does. The ideal rice preparation is with rice that is first aged for one year, freshly milled to remove about half or more of the bran and germ, and then soured. Since most of us cannot do this ourselves, our second best options are to choose between high quality white rice, and partially milled or brown rice prepared with a phytase-rich starter. The brown rice recipe is in the recipe section. If you are not going to soak your rice with a phytase-rich starter, then choose white rice.

Like the other grains, corn products should be fermented. There are many corn tortillas and other corn products in the stores that do not have the corn bran and germ. These should be low in phytic acid and not promote tooth decay. Just keep in mind if you eat any of these compromise foods that any unfermented grain eaten consistently has the potential to cause negative health effects in the long run.

**Calcium**—Just as in the Loetschental Valley grains go well with cheese. Calcium will block many negative effects from grains, nuts and beans. If you consume bread, have it with a large slice of cheese, or with a cup of raw milk, or both. Lentils go great with some yogurt on the side. The rickets-producing effect of oatmeal was limited by calcium.[172] When vitamin D is low in the diet, even phytic-acid-free grains can deplete levels of calcium.[173] This gives us an important clue to safe grain consumption: have calcium-containing foods with your grains.

**Vitamin C** —Vitamin C significantly counteracts the negative effects of grain anti-nutrients. Have vitamin C-rich foods with meals that have grains, nuts, beans or seeds in them. High quality unpasteurized dairy products have some vitamin C.

**Folic Acid** may play an important part in working with vitamin C to reduce the anti-nutritional effects of grains. High amounts of folic acid are found in liver from a variety of animals as well as in beans, spices, seaweed, leafy greens and asparagus.

## Vitamin C in Food

| Food 100 gram servings, about 3.5 ounces | Vitamin C Milligrams (mg) |
|---|---|
| Camu Camu | 2800 |
| Rose Hips | 2000 |
| Acerola Cherry | 1600 |
| Red Pepper | 190 |
| Parsley | 130 |
| Guava | 100 |
| Kiwi, Broccoli | 90 |
| Persimmon, Papaya, Strawberry | 60 |
| Orange | 50 |
| Kale | 41 |
| Lemon | 40 |
| Mandarin Orange, Tangerine, Raspberry | 30 |
| Raw Cabbage, Lime | 30 |
| Adrenal Gland | High |
| Calf Liver | 36 |
| Beef Liver | 31 |
| Oyster | 30 |
| Raw Milk 4 Cups | 19 |
| Lamb Brain | 17 |

**Vitamin D**—The anti-calcifying effects of whole grains are greatly reduced by vitamin D. Details about vitamin D were discussed in the last chapter. The more grains you consume, in particular oatmeal or whole grains, the more vitamin D your body needs. There is an upper limit to how much vitamin D will block the negative effect of whole grains. So even with plenty of cod liver oil, people consuming a high whole grain diet can have tooth decay problems. That is why it is important to consume grains that do not contain phytic acid or grain toxins. The combination of low phytic acid grains with vitamin D produced optimal bone growth and protection against rickets in diets that contained grains.

**Protein**—Traditional nut preparation combines roasted nuts with meat stews. Having protein with grains, nuts, seeds or beans may reduce some of their anti-nutritional characteristics.

· · · · · · · · · · · · · · · · · · · · · · · · · · · · · · · · · · · · · · · · · · · · · · · · · ·

**Summary of Basic Grain and Seed Consumption Guidelines**
Do not eat products containing whole grains or added bran.
Do not eat whole grains that are not home prepared.
Do not eat sprouted whole grain products.
Do not consume bleached white flour products.
Do not consume seeds regularly.
When you consume grains, nuts, seeds, or beans regularly, you
need to make sure to have adequate calcium, vitamin C and vita-
min D in your diet.

· · · · · · · · · · · · · · · · · · · · · · · · · · · · · · · · · · · · · · · · · · · · · · · · · ·

# Eating Grains At Home

**Introductory Guidelines**—If you are going to buy flour from the store, then
I recommend buying partially refined flour such as unbleached, unenriched
organic white flour. Do not use store-bought whole grain flour. Unbleached flour
is low in phytic acid. Just keep in mind that for the long run, eating only unsoured
unbleached flour is not an ideal health practice. Choose white basmati or white
jasmine or sushi rice for your homemade rice dishes.

· · · · · · · · · · · · · · · · · · · · · · · · · · · · · · · · · · · · · · · · · · · · · · · · · ·

**Bleached Flour vs. Unbleached Flour**
Unless labeled as unbleached, white flour has been subjected to
benzoyl peroxide or chlorine dioxide to make it appear bright
white. Many commercial flours add potassium bromate and are
also enriched. Choose unenriched organic unbleached white flour
when possible. Flour can go rancid easily, so flour that is freshly
ground will be healthier.

· · · · · · · · · · · · · · · · · · · · · · · · · · · · · · · · · · · · · · · · · · · · · · · · · ·

**Advanced Guidelines**—The indigenous practice all over the world is for grains
to be freshly ground before use. Many people have *Nourishing Traditions* by Sally
Fallon or other books which have many delicious recipes including whole grain
recipes. These recipes provide soaked and soured grain dishes that are easier to
digest. The careful suggestion I have is not to use whole grain flour. After you
fresh grind your whole grain you will want to sift it with a sifter or sieve to remove
the bran and germ. Then follow the recipe. You will have delicious dishes that are
easy to digest as a result. Grains that definitely require bran and germ removal
to be safe are corn, rye, spelt, kamut, barley, and wheat as well as grains directly
related to them. For rice you will need to decide if you want to use brown soaked
rice, partially milled soaked rice with the phytase starter, or white rice. If you can,
you will want to start with a vacuum sealed brown rice (since brown rice goes

easily rancid), remove about 50% of the bran, and then soak it with a phytase-rich starter as described in chapter six. Soured rice cakes will increase the vitality of the rice.

## Quinoa, and Buckwheat

I am not totally certain whether the grain bran or germ needs to be removed from the pseudo cereals of buckwheat and quinoa. Because I am unsure, if you eat the bran of these grains you do so at your own risk for exposure to plant toxins. If you want to eat these grains regularly, I suggest you do your own research.

## Grain Detoxification

When adults come to me with a difficult tooth that is not healing, I recommend they avoid grains for 2–3 weeks to let their body recover and find balance. Also avoid grains, nuts, beans and seeds temporarily if:

- You are eating a more nutrient-dense diet where you have achieved some cavity healing success, but not complete success, such as a once-painful tooth that now hurts occasionally.

- If you have been consuming whole grains that were not properly soured, or the bran from rye, kamut, spelt or wheat. It is possible that your intestinal lining is inflamed. Taking a temporary break from grains will help heal this problem.

After grain, nut, bean and seed detoxification you will more clearly be able to evaluate how grains are affecting your body, and which grains feel good for you to eat.

# Beans

Beans are high in phytic acid and lectins. Lathyrism is a disease attributed to poor people who in difficult environmental circumstances planted and consumed the extremely hardy bean *lathyrus sativus* (a type of sweet pea). The toxic substance that caused lathyrism is likely the toxic amino acid beta-N-oxalylamino-L-alanine. Its symptoms include walking difficulties, leg weakness and eventually complete paralysis. Other beans also contain quite a few plant toxins such as soy beans. Lima beans consumed in Nigeria as a staple involve a "painstaking processes" to make them safe to eat. [174]

To completely eliminate phytates, beans need to be soaked overnight in warm water, geminated for several days, and then soured. Most people will not be able to go through the lengths to remove all of the phytic acid in beans. Soaking beans overnight and then cooking them eliminates a good portion of phytic acid in smaller beans like lentils. Simply soaking beans overnight may be good enough for most people. Just boiling beans that are unsoaked will not remove a significant amount of phytic acid.

As with grains, different beans have different concentrations of plant toxins, and require different types of preparation methods. The exact details for indigenous cultures' preparation of commonly used beans are unobtainable by me at this time. But we can look at a few examples. In Latin America, beans are often fermented after the cooking process to make a sour porridge called chugo. In India lentils are typically consumed split. That means the outer layer, the husk, (equivalent to the bran in grains) is removed. Lentils without the bran are probably the safest beans to eat. Lentils can be soured into tasty cakes with rice called dosas. Take the same food combining precautions with beans as you would with grains. Eat beans with cheese, beans with vitamin D-containing-foods, and beans with vitamin C-rich vegetables and berries.

## Bean Suggestions

**Basic**
> Soak beans overnight and cook with kombu (sea vegetable) to soften them and aid digestion.
> Beans should be very soft and easy to digest when cooked.
> Choose smaller sized beans over larger ones.

**Advanced**
> Prepare soured beans in dishes like dosas.

# Breakfast Cereals and Granola

Breakfast cereals are manufactured at high temperatures. One study found that rats that ate only puffed wheat died before rats that were given no food at all. At least one breakfast cereal has killed lab rats faster than when the rats ate only the cardboard cereal box.[175] Many people unwisely continue to eat cold breakfast cereals because of the sugar-powered high it provides, and ignore the digestive distress that follows. Avoid the rancid and improperly prepared seeds, nuts and grains found in granolas, quick-rise breads and extruded breakfast cereals.

Many people eat store-bought granola, which is almost always unhealthy because of its high sugar content and high level of phytic acid from oats. Breakfast cereals, even when labeled organic, are not healthy foods. They contain few nutrients that your body can absorb. The sugar and flour combination will cause a rapid rise in blood sugar and thus promote tooth decay. The cartoon character on the cereal box does not really care if you or your child is healthy or not. Organic cereal may not have pesticides or additives, but it is not a nourishing food. If you must have cereal I suggest making soured homemade rice or hot rye cereal. Flour products need to be combined with protein, calcium, and fat.

# *Nuts and Nut Butters*

I read a comedic story of an indigenous group in the Amazon being introduced to peanut butter. They refused to eat it because it looked like human waste. Dogs are highly allergic to many types of nuts like walnuts and macadamia nuts. The symptoms that dogs suffer from nut poisoning include muscle tremors, seizures, vomiting, diarrhea, drooling, and elevated heart rate. As with grains, nuts are very high in plant toxins including phytic acid. The symptoms suffered by dogs that ingest nuts strongly suggest that nuts seem to have some substance, possibly lectins, which can affect the central nervous system. This nervous system effect is seen more clearly with dogs than with humans. Peanut allergies in humans can cause anaphylactic shock. This is just another potential sign of the potent plant toxins hidden in nuts. It is common for people with rampant tooth decay to rely on raw nut and seed butters as staples, including too much raw tahini.

Nuts are powerful inhibitors of iron absorption.[176] But phytic acid levels in nuts do not directly correlate with the decrease in iron absorption. Even though fresh coconut has a moderate amount of phytic acid, fresh coconut has little or no impact on iron absorption. Sprouting nuts improves iron absorption but only modestly. Vitamin C in the dose of 25 milligrams can prevent compounds in nuts from blocking iron absorption. Interestingly the iron-blocking characteristics of nuts may have to do with how nut proteins are digested.[177] This may explain the indigenous cultures' propensity to mix nuts with animal proteins.

## Phytic Acid Content of Nuts[178]

| Almond | Walnut | Peanut | Roasted Peanut | Sprouted Peanut | Hazel Nut | Brazil Nut |
|--------|--------|--------|----------------|-----------------|-----------|------------|
| 1.14   | 0.98   | 0.82   | 0.95           | 0.61            | 0.65      | 1.72       |

Just so you understand these figures, nuts contain about the same level of phytic acid as grains.

Do not misunderstand me; I think nuts are delicious—especially when they have been sprouted and low-temperature dehydrated, and then roasted to eliminate a large amount of phytic acid. It seems almost universal that indigenous cultures cooked their nuts in some way, such as adding them to meat soups and stews. The problem people have with nuts is that they are consuming too many raw, which means they are high in phytic acid, and too much as a staple, rather than as a part of a wholesome diet. An interesting note about macadamia nuts is that they are an aboriginal nut from Australia. Aboriginal peoples also had access to the highest vitamin C rich fruit on the planet, the kakadu plum. The high amounts of vitamin C in the aboriginal diet may have protected Australia's

Aborigines from plant toxins from macadamia nuts. Many types of macadamia nuts are known to be toxic and are not cultivated. A certain nut from Thailand needs to be buried in volcanic soil for 100 days, and then soaked for three days in water to make it safe to eat. Nuts contain nourishing vitamins, but also potent plant toxins that could adversely affect the central nervous system.

Since many people consume coconut flour, I will mention that dried coconut flour has about the same amount of phytic acid, 1.17 percent,[179]as many grains and other nuts. Coconut does not impact iron absorption which implies that it is much lower in the potent plant toxins found in grains and beans. Traditional societies shred coconut and usually cook it. This is not the same as commercially sold coconut flour. Coconut meal is a less powdered form of coconut flour. Coconut flour is made from the byproduct of coconut milk or coconut oil production. Coconut meal is usually used as animal feed. Even as an animal feed, its low protein digestibility causes pigs not to grow fully when it is used as a protein supplement.[180] It contains twice the fiber of the bran of grains. Because of the phytic acid content of coconut flour, consuming it regularly may affect your calcium / phosphorous metabolism. If you do consume coconut flour, make sure to have plenty of the vitamins and minerals that protect against phytic acid. Again, these are calcium, vitamin C, and fat-soluble vitamins A and D.

## Nut Suggestions

Nuts in moderation should not be a problem for most people with minor cavities. If you have severe tooth cavities, or have some nagging cavities that do not heal, consider avoiding nuts entirely until the problem resolves.

### Basic Guidelines

- Avoid commercially produced nut butters.
- Moderate the amount of nuts you eat; do not make them your staple food.
- Make sure to have plenty of food-based vitamin C, or calcium-rich foods with your nuts, such as roasted and skinless almonds with cheese.
- Be careful with almonds; they seem to be very high in plant toxins. The skins must be removed.

### Additional Intermediate Guidelines

- Only consume nuts, and nut butters made from them, that are soaked and dehydrated.

**Advanced Nut Guidelines**

- Roast nuts and use them for cooking, particularly with meat-based soups and stews.

- Extract the oil from freshly roasted nuts.

- Or, avoid nuts entirely.

# Trace Minerals Repair Cavities

The subject of trace minerals can get rather sticky since the utilization and balance of every mineral in our body is connected to all the other minerals in our body. I am not aware of any recognized minerals that are not important for our teeth. Minerals left out of the discussion here are still important. We have discussed the two essential minerals to remineralize teeth, calcium and phosphorus. Dentist and researcher Ralph Steinman recognized that magnesium, copper, iron, and manganese could all significantly influence tooth decay.

**Iron** deficiency is the most common nutrient deficiency in both less-developed as well as industrialized countries worldwide.[181] This deficiency is explained by the iron binding effects of phytic acid from grains and beans.

### Iron Content of Some Foods

| Food (100 gram servings, about 3.5 ounces) | Iron in Milligrams |
|---|---|
| beef / lamb spleen | 45 |
| duck / goose liver | 31 |
| clams | 12 |
| caviar | 12 |
| lamb kidneys | 12 |
| chicken / turkey liver | 12 |
| sun dried tomatoes | 9 |
| potatoes | 7 |
| parsley, raw | 6 |
| beef liver | 5 |

In general mollusks and organ meats are high in iron. Certain herbs like nettles are said to be high in iron. People eating diets containing grains are going to be much more susceptible to iron deficiencies due to the iron-binding qualities of phytic acid. Interestingly enough, cocoa powder is high in iron and copper.

This may explain people's addiction to chocolate, in particular people who do not eat meat.

**Copper** supports iron utilization in your body. Copper is the glue that holds tooth and bone together.[182] Liver and mollusks are high in copper. Mushrooms have small amounts of copper.

**Vitamins B$_{12}$ and folic acid** work together to help iron function properly in your body. Green leafy vegetables that are high in folate include asparagus, seaweed, spinach and okra. Animal sources of folate are clams, livers from a variety of animals, octopus, poultry giblets, kidneys, fish eggs and fish. I have found liver to be an almost magical cure for tooth decay. It is also a well known solution for anemia. Liver can be consumed cooked, seared or raw.

**Zinc** is necessary to produce enzymes and aids in controlling our blood sugar levels. Typically the factors inhibiting iron absorption such as phytic acid often have an even more pronounced negative effect on zinc absorption. Oysters are very high in zinc, with lesser amounts found in liver, red meats (beef, bison and lamb), shellfish, and turkey.

**Manganese** helps control blood sugar levels and aids in tooth mineralization.[183] Mussels, nuts, sweet potato, liver, kidney, blueberries, pineapple, and green and black tea, are more concentrated in their manganese content than other foods. Somewhat smaller amounts of manganese are present in most vegetables, berries, beans and sea foods. Phytic acid inhibits the absorption of manganese.

**Iodine** is helpful for fat metabolism and is found in sea foods, sea weeds, fish broth, butter, pineapple, artichokes, asparagus and dark green vegetables.

· · · · · · · · · · · · · · · · · · · · · · · · · · · · · · · · · · · · · · · · · · ·

### Liver Stops Cavities

Liver helps your body live. It contains nearly every vitamin and mineral needed to build healthy teeth and bones except for fat-soluble vitamin D, magnesium and calcium.

· · · · · · · · · · · · · · · · · · · · · · · · · · · · · · · · · · · · · · · · · · ·

# Do Multi-Vitamins Fight Tooth Decay?

Synthetic vitamins, and foods with synthetic vitamins added, offer little real benefit to your body. Synthetic vitamins are made with cheap substances and are not in a biochemical form that is easily absorbed by your body. As a result, most supplemental vitamins do little good and put quite a bit of internal stress on our organs. There is a reason why nature provides us with plant and animal food, and that we cannot live just by eating dirt or rocks. Our bodies view the synthetic vitamins as toxic substances that need to be rapidly eliminated. Hence the unusual odor or color of urine you may notice after consuming multi-vitamins. However when someone is very deficient in certain vitamins, even low quality vitamins can help. A stalk of celery or a serving of greens has more absorbable vitamins and minerals than a bottle of synthetic vitamin tablets.[184]

There are a handful of good vitamin supplements on the market. They will be made from whole foods. This keeps vitamins in a form that is recognizable and absorbable by your body. If you need to use a vitamin supplement, I recommend looking for a vitamin that does not have any type of sugar added, and a vitamin made as close to nature as possible using plants or herbs. Standard Process® makes many food-based nutritional supplements. They are generally not sold to the public but are available through many health care practitioners, particularly chiropractors and naturopathic doctors. One product from Standard Process® is called Bio-dent®. The ingredients include bovine adrenal, bovine spleen, bone meal and calcium lactate. I have seen amazing results with this vitamin, but unfortunately not everyone gets excellent results with it.

There are other trace mineral supplements from the land and the sea. One example is shilajit which is an asphalt-like, mineral-rich pitch, or tar. Fulvic mineral deposits are from plant life that has been broken down millions of years ago. Consult with your health care practitioner to discover if these are right for you.

# Soy Products

A friend of mine thought eating large portions of tofu was a good idea. In a short time her hair began falling out and her skin turned pale. Soy contains plant hormones that need to be disabled through a careful fermentation process, which tofu does not undergo. High levels of phytic acid in soy reduce the assimilation of calcium, magnesium, copper, iron and zinc. Phytic acid in soy is not neutralized by ordinary preparation methods such as soaking, sprouting, and long, slow cooking. High phytate diets have caused growth problems in children.[185] Fermented soy products, such as special fermented soy drinks (not available in the store), natural soy sauce, miso and tempeh can be acceptable. However, use fermented soy with care and awareness.

## Fake Milks

**Soy milk** contains enzyme inhibitors and excess estrogen. I have read of a fermented soy drink that can cure cancer, but this is not the same as the cheap, denatured, anti-nutrient-rich and overly processed soy products sold in grocery stores.

Store-bought **rice milk** and other nut milks may contain large amounts of grain and nut anti-nutrients like phytic acid. Although it may not say it on the label, rice bran may be the main ingredient of some rice milks.

**Nut and seed milks** may also contain high concentrations of plant toxins.

Nuts are highly prized by native groups for their oils, and can be made at home. Yet homemade milks may contain highly potent anti-nutrients or plant toxins if they are not thoroughly cooked.

If you are a rice milk or nut milk lover, make it at home yourself. Use recipes that use cooked ingredients, or involve heating or fermentation. Do not settle for cheap imitations.

# Nightshades

Tomatoes, potatoes (but not sweet potatoes or yams), eggplant, goji berries, and peppers of every sort fall into the nightshade category. Nightshades contain calcitrol. The amount of calcitrol varies for each particular nightshade. Calcitrol is a hormone that signals our body to use calcium from our diet and it can easily lead to too much blood calcium,[186] thus calcitrol can imbalance our calcium to phosphorous blood ratio. This can easily lead to tooth decay.[187] Symptoms of too much blood calcium can include tooth decay on top of the teeth, or excess calculus deposits. Too much calcitrol from nightshades can also lead to calcium deposits in the body. This is one reason why nightshades have been connected with chronic pain or inflammation such as joint or back pain. The effects of nightshades may be canceled by other foods in your diet such as calcium, or vitamin D, but I am not certain. If you are struggling with tooth decay and cannot seem to stop it, then try taking nightshades out of your diet.

## Potatoes

White potatoes typically contain moderate amounts of phytic acid.[188] They are members of the nightshade family. White potatoes can be included in a diet that will prevent cavities. They are not crucial to remove from your diet, but for some people, removing the potato might make the key difference. Due to their nightshade characteristics potatoes may in some way contribute to tooth decay in an imbalanced diet.

A better alternative to modern potatoes are yams and sweet potatoes. Sweet potatoes do not contain any of the anti-nutrient phytic acid.[189] Yams contain a small amount of phytic acid. The only problem with sweet potatoes or yams is that they may be too sweet for individuals with blood sugar sensitivities. Taro root and yucca (cassava) contain a significant amount of phytic acid. [190] This may explain why some cultures ferment these roots or convert them into beer. By and large, sweet potatoes, yams, or other tubers like taro root, and yucca are excellent staples to include in a healthy tooth-decay-prevention diet. They go together marvelously well with fats and proteins.

# *Organic Food Is Better*

Whenever possible, go for organic food. I am not talking about packaged food here. I am talking about wholesome unprocessed meat, fruit and vegetables. Published studies show that pesticides do show up in children's bodies and bloodstreams soon after consuming pesticide-ridden conventional foods.[191] It is wrong that our culture allows poisons to be sprayed on our food. The good news is that you do not have to eat organic foods to be immune to tooth decay. That bad news is that pesticides put an unnecessary strain on the body and they may lead to other health problems. There is also a wide range of organically approved pesticides. While they are better than other pesticides, there are still many malignant substances sprayed on organic food. I recommend doing whatever you can to support small and local farms such as going to farmer's markets, or shopping at stores that buy from local farms. This is not a requirement, but something feels good about buying food from and supporting the small family farm.

## Healthy Fats

Healthy fats support smooth hormonal function and are a great source of energy. They come from organic sources and include avocado, palm and coconut oil, olive oil, butter, beef, pork, chicken, and duck fat. Conventional vegetable oils are not healthy fats. Animal fats contain special vitamins that remineralize teeth, while vegetable fats generally do not.

### *Dangerous Fats*

**Trans fats** —*Trans* fats come from adding hydrogen to vegetable oil through a process called hydrogenation. Margarine is an example of a *trans* fat. Factory made *trans* fats are toxic to the body.[192] *Trans* fats have replaced real fats like organic butter, tallow and lard. Eating *trans* fats means you have replaced important fat-soluble vitamins from animal fats with man made toxic fats.

    **Canola Oil** —Canola is not the name of a plant, but rather a shorted term for Canadian Oil. The FDA prohibits the use of canola oil in baby formulas because it retards growth.[193] The *trans* fat content of canola oil is listed at 0.2 percent, yet independent research has found *trans* levels as high as 4.6 percent in commercial liquid oil.[194] Canola oil is extracted by a combination of high temperature mechanical pressing and solvent extraction. My experience in consuming canola oil is that it makes me feel congested and I start coughing. Because it is cheap, and believed to be healthy due to its monosaturated fat content, canola oil is what many restaurants and health food stores unfortunately use for frying their food. If they only knew that this rancid oil was not good for their customers they might stop using it. These establishments falsely tout the health benefits of canola oil. The inferior taste and feeling from foods cooked in canola oil repels me, and probably many customers from these food establishments.

## Nut and Seed Oils

Nut and seed oils have been a part of the human diet for a very long time. Walnut oil is popular in France and Italy. For the nut oils to be healthy, many of them require careful processing, or fresh pressing. Limit or avoid nut and seed oils as best you can unless they are from small artisan producers.

**Safflower, soy and corn oils** are all on the list of oils to avoid. Because of their delicate structure these vegetable oils are especially dangerous after being heated in the process of cooking or frying.[195]

# Hidden Monosodium Glutamate

Consuming unnatural forms of monosodium glutamate (MSG) may alter your endocrine gland balance. This can disrupt your body's ability to regulate the homeostasis required to allow your parotid gland to send signals for your teeth to remineralize. Viewed from this perspective, MSG may be a contributing factor in tooth decay. Most store-bought soups, sauces and broth mixes contain MSG. MSG shows up secretly in product labels under different names. Avoid products containing the following ingredients: Hydrolyzed Vegetable Protein (HVP), Textured Protein, Yeast Extract, Autolyzed Plant Protein, and anything with the word glutamate, or glutamic.

## Sweet Drinks

Health food stores are loaded with sweetened and protein-fortified vegetable and fruit juices. Most of these products are pasteurized and therefore skeletonized foods. Avoid pasteurized vegetable and fruit juices. Sweet drinks from the store are loaded with sugar. They provide empty calories and are not a part of a healthy diet. Here and there a naturally sweetened drink will not do you much harm if you do not have cavities. But these foods are not for people trying to stop tooth decay. Watch out in particular for sports drinks and sweetened tea. Replace these with unsweetened tea, raw milk, whey or kefir.

Kombucha is a popular health tonic. It has a wonderful array of nutrients and probiotics. While it is a great beverage, I recommend people who are trying to stop cavities to avoid it. Typically kombucha available commercially has a sugar content that is too high, as not all of the sugar has been digested by the bacteria and yeast organisms. Just to be clear, kombucha, especially home-made or the equivalent where most of the sugar is fermented is a life-promoting drink. It just does not work well if you are trying to stop tooth decay.

# *Health Food Bars, Energy Bars and Tooth Decay*

Health food bars have made national news headlines for their ability to cause tooth decay. People who have never had a cavity in their adult teeth all of a sudden have several large ones.[196] I have talked with many people who developed large cavities rapidly, or who have chipped teeth as a result of health food bar consumption. The culprit here is not bacteria or the sticky gooeyness of the bars. The problem with the nutrition bars is the ingredients. Many health food bars have a rancid taste which is covered up by copious amounts of sugar. Health food bars typically contain multiple ingredients you will find on our "foods to avoid" lists. The combination of isolated protein fragments, high intensity sweeteners, and unprocessed whole grains chock full of phytic acid in health food bars creates a potent recipe for tooth bone loss, otherwise known as tooth decay.

## Addictive Substances

Too much coffee consumption and not enough protein lead to a decrease in bone density.[197] Caffeine stimulates the adrenal glands to release an adrenaline-like substance. This substance causes the liver to release sugar into the blood.[198] Caffeine will cause alterations in your calcium / phosphorous balance and over-stimulate your glandular system. People typically rely on caffeine to cover up a sense of depletion. Eating high quality saturated fats, like butter, coconut oil, or animal fats will help restore the balance of energy metabolism.

Alcohol consumption is connected with bone loss. In a small survey, moderate or heavy beer drinkers seem to develop cavities. Beer and wine can cause cavities because of the grains or the grain sugar in the alcohol, or the alcohol itself. Alcohol consumption raises blood sugar, and depletes the body of magnesium, zinc, manganese potassium and folic acid.[199] The quality and type of alcohol makes a difference as well. Naturally fermented alcoholic drinks like ancient beer or homemade apple cider may have beneficial effects on the body when the alcohol content is not high. That being said, if you want to heal your cavities, then it is best to moderate and/or eliminate alcohol consumption. Distilled liquors need to be avoided. Wine and unpasteurized beers appear to be acceptable when used in moderation if you do not have significant cavities. In excess, wine and beer are overtaxing to the liver. Regular consumption of commercially brewed beers will contribute to cavities.

Chocolate is high in iron and other trace minerals. It is also is usually paired with significant amounts of sugar. The sugar mixed with the chocolate will contribute to tooth decay. Cocoa powder is extremely high in phytic acid and tannins (an anti-nutrient).[200] To stop tooth decay, chocolate consumption should be greatly limited or eliminated. Healthy people can eat moderate amounts of chocolate and not have tooth decay. The most ancient preparation of chocolate is a fermentation process that converts the chocolate into beer.

Sugar is a highly addictive drug-like substance in our modern diet. While a little bit of natural sugar is safe to eat, too much sugar produces a numbing effect. Too much sugar can offer a glimpse of pleasure and a feeling of relaxation in an otherwise stressful life. Some people feel justified in the excess intake of stimulating substances because of the pain-numbing euphoria it can produce.

## Prescription Drugs, Recreational Drugs and Your Teeth

Drugs, including over-the-counter medications usually alter your glandular system and will affect your calcium and phosphorous ratios. Prescription and recreational drugs, along with cigarettes, may alter your body's ability to utilize nutrients from food. Many people in the western world have lost their ability to digest and utilize fat and protein due to damage caused by western drugs.

Maverick physician Dr. Henry Bieler, author of the bestselling *Food Is Your Best Medicine*, wrote:

> *As a practicing physician for over fifty years, I have reached three basic conclusions as to the cause and cure of disease.*
>
> *The first is that the primary cause of disease is not germs.*
>
> *The second conclusion is that in almost all cases the use of drugs in treating patients is harmful. Drugs often cause serious side effects, and sometimes even create new diseases. The dubious benefits they afford the patient are at best temporary.*
>
> *My third conclusion is that disease can be cured through the proper use of correct foods.*[201]

Many western drugs over-stimulate our glands, poison our livers, and produce the illusion of health. The long-term effects of many drugs are not known. They rarely offer long-term cures for diseases because the cause of disease is never addressed. These assertions are also directed towards the use of vaccinations. Documented evidence has shown that vaccines cause disease. Vaccines will be discussed more thoroughly in the children's tooth decay section. Birth control pills increase one's risk of developing gum disease, which illustrates how hormones and medications can alter our mineral metabolism.[202]

Many recreational drugs also cause harm to our bodies. While prescription drugs usually aim to treat symptoms of physical disease, recreational drugs are used to numb people overwhelmed by emotional distress. Recreational drugs add a stimulating way to give relief to emotional pain that people feel. Like prescription drugs, regular use of recreational drugs does not cure the problem, but rather puts off dealing with life. Drugs for recreation are not in harmony with Nature's laws and principles.

## *Thanks Giving*

Together we have just looked at some of the best and some of the worst of foods modern society has to offer. Too many processed and refined foods will lead to diseases and tooth decay. This was illustrated by Weston Price's photographs and research. Seeing the problems in the foods you may be eating can be challenging. Here I just want to give thanks for having food. Whether it is good or not, I am thankful that I have enough food to eat. Many people in the world do not even have the luxury of choosing their daily menu. Giving thanks for our food is a way to honor and respect Nature's gifts. When the positive vibration of thankfulness fills our lives and our culture, we will no longer have foods that will destroy our health.

*Chapter 5*

# Nutrition Protocols that Remineralize and Repair Cavities

**Hippocrates believed in *vis medicatrix naturae*—**Nature's innate ability to heal. Weston Price also acknowledged this same principle, concluding that "Life in all its fullness is this mother nature obeyed."[203] All you need to do to heal cavities is understand Nature's rules for health, and then follow them. When you follow these rules, the built-in ability for your teeth to heal will take over. Dr. Price's tooth decay prevention protocol has shown a success rate of over 90%.[204] To heal your teeth, align yourself with this subtle natural force, and change how you eat.

## *Nature's Rules for Healing Teeth*

Let us review some key points of the book thus far to help you align with and understand the principles that govern the functions of your body and teeth:

- Tooth decay is caused by environmental forces such as food; you have complete control over your diet.

- "Dangerous" bacteria are not the cause of cavities and do not randomly attack innocent victims.

- Our modern diet is deficient in fat-soluble vitamins and minerals needed for healthy teeth and bones.

- Tooth decay occurs when your body chemistry falls out of balance and your body sends hormonal signals that tell your teeth to stop remineralizing. The imbalance is caused by blood sugar spikes and a disruption in your calcium and phosphorous metabolism. Eating plenty of vegetables, limiting your sugar intake, eating enough proteins and a diet that includes plenty of fat-soluble vitamins usually resolves this imbalance.

- Dentists are surgeons who treat the symptoms of dental disease with surgery. Dental treatments usually provide only short term results. Dentistry has never promised to remineralize cavities or to prevent future cavities.

# *Remineralize Your Teeth with Diet*

In the previous chapter I presented detailed dietary instructions on what to eat and why in order to remineralize your carious teeth. We learned about Nature's health principles by examining the diets of indigenous peoples across the globe. I will now compile several highly effective dietary programs based upon decades of research performed by some of the world's best dentists including Weston Price and Melvin Page. I will also draw upon the lifetime of dental experience of dentist George Heard, and the decades of controlled feeding experiments by doctors Edward and May Mellanby. In addition these programs are brought together using volumes of research from dental and nutritional publications as well as from my personal experience of five years in helping people remineralize their teeth with diet.

Each program presented here may have new tips, tricks and ideas for you to learn. You will also find meal ideas and recipes in the next chapter. Nothing in this chapter is meant to replace your innate knowledge. If something does not feel right, or does not work for you, then please change these guidelines to fit what feels the best for you. I will offer a basic program that is easiest to follow, a balanced program designed for most readers, and an advanced as well as a vegetarian program.

Each program involves several important aspects to heal tooth decay. I want you to understand the structure so you can create the type of diet you want.

1. Add fat-soluble vitamins A, D and Activator X to the diet.

2. Consume portions of protein throughout the day to balance blood sugar.

3. Avoid or reduce modern denatured foods.

4. Eat foods to increase mineral intake, particularly broth, dairy products and vegetables.

For simplicity's sake I will consistently recommend Green Pasture's™ products in these programs. You can use the guidelines in chapter two to find substitute sources of fat-soluble vitamins to your liking. Green Pasture's™ products can be purchased at: **codliveroilshop.com**

# Balanced Tooth Decay
# Remineralizing Program

## Food Intake Suggestions

½ teaspoon two or three times per day of Green Pasture's™ Blue Ice™ Royal Blend

2–4 cups of raw, whole-fat dairy per day in the form of milk, kefir, whey, yogurt, clabber, or buttermilk. You can substitute about two ounces of cheese for every cup of fluid dairy. Also consider an eggnog smoothie as described in the next chapter.

2–4 ounces of raw cheese

1–2 cups of homemade gelatin-rich bone broth per day from any animal including beef, chicken, and fish.

6–18 ounces of high quality animal protein throughout the day and prepared for maximum digestion including stews, or raw, seared or marinated variations. Beef, chicken, pork, fish, lamb, eggs and so on. Have some protein with every meal. Divide your ideal weight by 15 for your minimum daily protein requirement in ounces.

Plenty of cooked vegetables including but not limited to beet greens, kale, chard, zucchini, broccoli, celery, and string beans. These can be consumed as soups. I provide a mineral-rich recipe for an Ayurvedic Green Drink in the next chapter.

At least once per day have something fermented such as kefir, yogurt or sauerkraut.

1 teaspoon or more of healthy fat with every meal. The fat can be raw or cooked. Grass-fed butter or ghee is preferred. Other animal fats like lard or tallow are also good choices.

Twice per week eat a comfortable amount of liver from any animal.

Twice per week choose one shellfish or other organ of land animals. Here are some suggestions:

Oysters, clams, crab or lobster (consumed with innards), whole crayfish

Fish eggs

1–3 tablespoons of bone marrow

Animal tongue or kidneys from any animal

You might want more carbohydrates in this type of diet. If you need more see if sweet potatoes or yams work for you. You may also use phytate-free grains like sourdough bread made from unbleached flour (bran and germ removed). If your diet includes grains that are soured to remove phytates, please review the grains section in the previous chapter to make sure you are using grains mindfully.

## Foods to Avoid in All Protocols

Even with a healthy diet, some foods on this list will cause a tooth disaster. Other foods may not be that bad for your teeth if consumed on occasion. The details on these foods were discussed in the previous chapter. The more you avoid these foods, the more completely your teeth can remineralize.

I have received some complaints that the food protocols presented in the previous edition of this book are too strict or complicated to follow. My job is to share with you my best understanding of Nature's principles for health so that you can activate your body's natural tooth and gum healing abilities. Please do not interpret this as me dictating to you what you can and cannot eat. You are always free to do whatever you want with your life including eating foods that can be toxic to your body. If you cannot follow the recommendations on this list, or believe that I have made mistakes, or feel that you deserve to eat foods on the "avoid" list, then know that such a decision may affect your ability to heal your teeth. The more disciplined you are in avoiding foods that cause or aggravate deficiency states in your body the more successful you will be in healing cavities quickly. How you translate that teaching into action is totally your choice. I suggest giving these guidelines your best attempt, and then judge how you feel.

**Avoid sweets and foods sweetened with these items**—white sugar, cane sugar, evaporated cane juice, xylitol, agave nectar, jams, dried fruit, candy bars, health food bars, yacon syrup, erythritol, lo han, palm sugar, coconut sugar, stevia extract, glycerin, fructose, high fructose corn syrup, inulin, fructooligosaccharides (FOS), brown rice syrup, malted barley and grain sweeteners, maltodextrin, sucrose, dextrose, sucralose, aspartame, and saccharine. If you do not know what the sweetener is then avoid it.

**Acceptable sweets**—Unheated honey, organic maple syrup (grade B preferred), real cane sugar (Heavenly Organics™ or Rapunzel's), stevia (actual herb only; no stevia extracts), whole fruit including dates or fresh squeezed fruit juice but not fruit extracts or concentrates.

**Avoid white flour or denatured grain products including organically labeled ones:** crackers, cookies, doughnuts, pies, breakfast cereals, granola, muffins, pastries, flour tortillas, bagels, noodles, pasta, pizza, couscous, bread that is organic but not made from freshly ground and fermented grains, and nearly every packaged product that contains grain products. Watch out for sprouted whole grain products and gluten-free foods made with brown rice.

**Avoid whole grains** that are not soured according to guidelines presented in this chapter including whole wheat, rye, kamut, spelt, brown rice, and quinoa.

**Acceptable grains**—Sourdough bread made with unbleached flour (bran and germ removed), partially milled rice that is soaked with a starter (white rice is acceptable), grains properly soured based upon indigenous preparation methods.

**Avoid raw nuts and nut butters** —including all raw nuts, as well as peanut butter, raw almond butter and raw tahini.

**Acceptable nuts and butters** —Nuts and nut butters should be roasted or otherwise cooked. Low temperature dehydrated nuts and nut butters are acceptable in moderation.

**Avoid hydrogenated oils** —such as margarine or other butter substitutes.

**Avoid low quality vegetable oils** —such as vegetable, soybean, canola, corn and safflower oils. Avoid potato chips, Crisco®, and any food not fried in a natural fat. Unfortunately most restaurants use these cheap vegetable cooking oils which make their food unhealthy for regular consumption.

**Acceptable fats** —are all natural, organic and ideally from small producers. They include coconut oil, palm oil, olive oil, butter, lard, tallow, chicken, duck and goose fat.

**Avoid pasteurized, homogenized or grain-fed milk and ice cream.** Also avoid low-fat dairy products and powdered milk along with anything that contains it.

**Avoid store-bought rice milk, soy milk and nut milks like hemp and almond.**

**Acceptable dairy products are raw and grass-fed from any type of ruminant** and whole fat, not skimmed.

**When you have only grocery store options for dairy products** —then choose pasteurized, but grass-fed dairy products from smaller producers. Yogurt, butter and grass-fed cheese that are pasteurized are the best of the pasteurized dairy products. There are some nice pasteurized grass-fed cheeses from Australia, Ireland and New Zealand that are reasonable in cost.

**Avoid table salt**—Many foods have commercial, refined salt added. Table salt seems highly irritating to the body.

**Acceptable salts**—Himalayan salt, Celtic Sea Salt®, and other sea salts are good to use. Celtic Sea Salt® seems the best out of these options.

**Avoid conventional fast foods and junk foods** —These foods are usually high in *trans* fats, food additives and sugar.

**Avoid stimulants**—Do not drink coffee, sweetened drinks, sports drinks, or alcohol. Do not smoke cigarettes. Reduce or avoid chocolate.

**Avoid unfermented soy** including isolated soy protein, tofu, soy / veggie burgers, soy "meat" and soymilk.

**Acceptable soy products are traditionally fermented**—You can have small amounts of unpasteurized soy sauce, miso, and natto.

**Avoid green powders** —most green powder supplements have sugar added and contain questionable ingredients. There are a few exceptions to this rule, which would be 100% food-based dried powders with no sweeteners added.

**Avoid factory farmed meat, fish, and eggs.** These offer inferior quality proteins.

**Acceptable proteins are grass-fed or wild**. These offer superior quality and bolster health.

**Avoid too much fruit.** Even though fruit is natural, people often eat too much. Be very careful with sweet fruits like as oranges, bananas, grapes, peaches, blueberries and pineapple.

**Avoid prescription drugs, over-the-counter drugs, and vaccines**. These alter your glandular balance and many are causative factors in tooth decay.

**Avoid food additives** like MSG, nitrates, and nitrites.

**Avoid commercially processed foods, such as TV dinners and packaged saucc mixes.**

**Avoid synthetic vitamins and any foods containing them.**

# The "One-Amazing-Meal-a-Day" Protocol

This is a useful introductory protocol for people who want to make a good dent against tooth decay (pun intended), but who have difficulty instituting a complete dietary overhaul. How well your teeth remineralize is a factor of the mineral and fat-soluble vitamin density of your diet, along with the avoidance of foods that deplete your body of nutrients. This program is designed for someone who is very busy, does not like to prepare his own food, or in other situations when it is too difficult to have three or more solid meals per day. This program is not recommended for people who have severe cavities, tooth infections, or who are trying to heal highly sensitive teeth. This program will not be as effective as the balanced program, but it will be effective for most people who want to prevent cavities, or heal small cavities naturally. This program is based on Weston Price's one-good-meal-per-day diet for poor children that we described in chapter two. The goal of this program is to get most of your daily supply of vitamins and minerals from one superlative meal. In the other meals of the day you will need to watch out for the foods that cause the most havoc on your teeth, but you will be able to eat a wide variety of foods that are convenient for you. Reduce to the best of your ability other foods on the just-mentioned "avoid" list.

## Food Intake Suggestions

½ teaspoon two or three times per day of Green Pasture's™ Blue Ice™ Royal Blend

2 cups of grass-fed, whole-fat raw milk, kefir, clabber, or yogurt or 4 ounces of raw grass-fed cheese. For non-dairy alternatives you will need about 3 cups of a variety of cooked green vegetables.

Nourishing meat and/or fish stew made with a gelatin-rich broth prepared by simmering animal bones. Many of the ingredients listed below can be included in your stew.

2-8 ounces of high-quality land or sea protein.

Vitamin C-rich foods such as broccoli, cauliflower, bell peppers, mustard greens, cabbage, sauerkraut, kohlrabi, liver and adrenal glands.

Plenty of other vegetables.

Twice per week choose one shellfish or other organ of land animals to include with your meals. Examples:

Oysters, clams, crab or lobster (consumed with innards), whole crayfish

Fish eggs

Bone marrow added to your soup, or liver, animal tongue or kidneys from any animal

If you cannot have a meat or fish stew, you will want to have a cup gelatin-rich bone broth on the side with tender cuts of your favorite meats, or rich seafoods. Have plenty of healthy fats with your meals.

During your other meals you will need to avoid foods that are especially harmful to your teeth including highly sweetened drinks, foods with high fructose corn syrup or other high intensity sweeteners, whole grains that are not thoroughly soured, oatmeal, breakfast cereals and soy products. If you choose to eat bread, make it sourdough whenever possible. Choose white rice (or white rice products), or partially milled rice over brown rice (or brown rice products) in this introductory program since brown rice takes more care to disable the substantial amounts of phytic acid it contains. Consider replacing sweetened desserts with fruit.

## *Tips for Going out to Eat*

Many of us go out to eat, especially those of you who are busy and will be following the one-amazing-meal-a-day plan. The minimal goal of restaurant eating is to enjoy nourishing and tasty foods that will not set you back in your tooth or gum healing process. The restaurants that are thoroughly engaged in whole-food, nutrient-dense cooking with high quality ingredients tend to be the most expensive. The style of their cuisine typically has at least some inspiration from traditional French cooking. These restaurants do not use excess grains to fill you up with low-cost calories, and you can expect local ingredients, grass-fed meats, and wild caught fish. Many of them understand the value of organ meats and serve sweetbreads, liver, oysters and clams. Expect to pay $20-30 or considerably more per adult. I recommend that you avoid pasta or grain-based dishes from these restaurants. If you are the type of person who can afford to dine this way regularly, why not take care of yourself and give your body what it needs by eating at the best restaurants?

Before going to restaurants I usually look at the menu to see if there is some type of high-quality protein such as a wild caught fish, or grass-fed meat. Restaurants offering catfish, tilapia, shrimp, and salmon are usually serving the farm-raised variety. Most of the other types of fish in restaurants are usually wild caught. We also call restaurants in advance to see what type of cooking oil they use. Some restaurants cook food by smoking or grilling, in which case the cooking oil becomes much less of an issue. Depending on the dish or restaurant you might be able to request that your food be fried in butter or lard, as compared with the unhealthy vegetable oil too many restaurants use. We avoid deep fried dishes fried in vegetable oil. Do not be afraid to sneak your favorite butter into the restaurant.

Many restaurants try to fill you up on bread. I generally avoid this bread although my family will eat a piece or two if they are hungry. If you are getting a sandwich or a hamburger, try to get it on sourdough bread. If the bread is not sourdough, consider eating only half of the bread served.

When you go out to eat while you are trying to heal your teeth, I would encourage you to skip the sweet drinks, beer, wine and desserts on the menu; all of these items will affect your body chemistry adversely. With a little bit of discipline you can convert your restaurant adventures into meals that support or at least do not harm your efforts to heal your tooth decay.

# *Advanced Tooth Decay Healing*

This diet is good for people trying to turn around severe tooth problems. Every item in this diet is designed to be the best of the best in terms of food nutrient density and in its ability to remineralize teeth extremely fast. This regime also aims to capture elements of a diet that may be close to optimal in maintaining health. Following these recommendations will make your teeth rock hard. Even if this diet is not right for you, or if it seems unbalanced, you can take aspects from this framework and add it to your personal tooth remineralizing diet. Please prepare the food or pick and choose items from this list so that you feel your efforts are life-affirming based upon your belief systems and personal goals. In this diet you want all your protein to be as fresh as possible. The highest quality proteins are seafoods and meats that have never been frozen. If it is so fresh that is has never been refrigerated, then all the better.

## Daily Food Intake

½ teaspoon two or three times per day of Green Pasture's™ Blue Ice™ Royal Blend

⅛ teaspoon two or three times per day Blue Ice™ fermented skate liver oil

2 ounces of grass-fed liver four or more days per week. Raw is preferred but cooked or seared with onions is totally fine.

4–12 oysters, clams or mussels several times per week. Raw is preferred, cooked is acceptable.

1–2 tablespoons of bone marrow cooked or raw several times per week.

2–8 cups of fermented dairy per day such as kefir, yogurt, whey, buttermilk or clabber. 0–4 ounces of raw cheese depending on how much dairy you consume.

1–2 tablespoons of raw cream several times per week.

8 or more ounces of protein from grass-fed or wild sources per day. Proteins are to be consumed raw, rare, or fermented such as ceviche, or as a stew.

Ideally your proteins should be a mix of land foods and sea foods.

1–2 cups of fish head soup per day. Otherwise use beef, chicken and so forth.

2–4 raw eggs. These can be consumed in smoothies with your soured milk. Alternatively have your eggs soft boiled.

Fermented vegetables like sauerkraut

Cooked leafy green vegetables or vegetable soup. If you are a primal food eater then vegetable juice is fine.

Bonus items to this diet include: Colostrum, fish eggs, crab and lobsters with the innards, spring and summer yellow butter, organ meats like adrenal, thyroid and the brain, and animal blood. Eat the crab and lobsters cooked, some of the glands are best raw and the brain should be cooked.

In this diet carbohydrates are obtained mostly from dairy products. If you are not trying to heal severe cavities, and you are not on a low-carb program then you can add sourdough bread from unbleached flour made from freshly ground and sifted grains (bran and germ removed). Alternatively you can include sweet potatoes, yams, and other root vegetables. Souring or fermenting these vegetables will enhance their digestibility.

If you do not have cavities, then an ideal diet can include moderate amounts of lacto-fermented drinks and homemade alcohols that do not contain malted grains or commercial yeasts such as sweet potato beer, apple cider allowed to ferment, grapes allowed to ferment or homemade mead (honey wine).

People following this diet must strictly avoid all processed and denatured food. Generally the highest quality ingredients are obtained directly from the farm, such as through buyers clubs or farmers' markets.

# Healing Tooth Cavities on a Vegetarian Diet

I created the vegetarian program because it is possible to significantly improve your dental health as a vegetarian. Even though I do not recommend anyone to choose vegetarianism as a way of life, I want to respond to the many requests for help from vegetarians. I ask you to reflect on a few points before continuing onto the vegetarian program. Just to be clear in this discussion, when I say meat, it includes fish. If you want to avoid land animal food and only consume sea food, then you can use the other protocols in this book and enjoy very gratifying results.

When I was a vegetarian I never completely thought through why I had chosen that lifestyle, although I believed I did not want to contribute to the killing of animals. Instead I slowly and unknowingly started to kill myself by consuming large amounts of tofu to satisfy my hunger. My two years of vegetarianism ended when I was on a vision quest. High up on Mount Shasta in California I fasted for two nights and three days. I could not finish the last night of the vision quest because I became obsessed with one vision only: a turkey sandwich! I was starving and depleted and I resolved during that fast to quit vegetarianism. I no longer am vegetarian and I do not encourage a vegetarian diet for women who are pregnant or planning for pregnancy, or who are breastfeeding. Neither do I encourage a vegetarian diet for children.

Current commercial livestock practices around the world damage the environment, and the animals are in general mistreated. But depriving ourselves of what we need by avoiding animal foods sends out into the world the energy of impoverishment and deprivation. I did not realize that there was a choice of animals humanely cared for. There are even some grass-fed farms that include prayers in a ceremony before killing the animal. By choosing foods carefully, making certain that the animals are well cared for and raised humanely, I personally feel it is good to satisfy my body's hunger by eating meat.

In an idealized world, I probably would not eat meat because I honestly prefer not to kill things. Yet until that idealized world becomes a reality, I do not have energy or vibrancy without eating some type of animal protein with every meal. Healthy vegetarians still need animal fats and proteins; they simply get them from dairy products and eggs. Before domestication of animals, humans hunted their animal proteins. Nature's design for humans, who are able to fashion tools, is clearly for us to hunt. Humans would not be able to live in colder climates without making clothing from animal skins. Our genetic and ancestral heritage is one of hunting and gathering.

Most people are vegetarian for religious purposes. Over the last millennium or two, certain groups relied upon a meat-free diet to aid them on their spiritual path. Today many monks and spiritual leaders eat some animal meat; they just do not kill it themselves. So until the wolf and the lamb feed together and lions start eating only grass, I am going to continue to eat and recommend that people eat some type of animal flesh.

There are healthy vegetarian societies in the world, but this is not a common finding. When Weston Price did his field studies he could not locate even one traditional culture that was vegetarian. However Dr. Price did not travel to India. Village people in certain parts of India, following a carefully designed diet based upon ancient Ayurvedic knowledge, have what appears to be a low rate of tooth decay. Each part of their diet is carefully orchestrated including planting and harvesting in harmony with the moon cycles, special soil fertility practices, special combinations of vegetables to ensure mineral balance, absolutely no processed food of any sort, grains aged for one year and freshly ground, aged sugar, special spices to enhance digestion, herbs and berries such as amalaki to enhance the mineral content of diet, complete avoidance of all nightshades, and perhaps the most potent and nutrient-dense dairy on the planet from the water-buffalo. The milk is also processed differently in accordance with the season. A rare few deeply spiritual and traditionally rooted societies have found ways to create enough mineral density in their diet to have a high resistance to tooth decay without relying upon animal flesh. This type of diet is very difficult to recreate in the United States.

The key problem area for the vegetarian diet is fat-soluble vitamin D which is the most important fat-soluble vitamin for remineralizing teeth. Even most grass-fed milk is low in fat-soluble vitamin D. It is highly likely that special foods given to the water-buffalo and its ability to absorb and utilize sunlight led to milk with fairly high vitamin D content. Since I know for certain that Green Pasture's™ X-Factor Gold™ high vitamin butter oil is rich in vitamin D, (most butters are not rich in vitamin D, even many grass-fed variants) using this regularly is an essential key for a vegetarian plan to work well. To purchase it go to: **codliveroilshop.com**

The vegetarian plan relies heavily on minerals from vegetables. People who eat meat and fish can get some missing dietary minerals from animal flesh. On the vegetarian plan there is not going to be that extra measure of safety. Success will be partially dependent on the quality and freshness of the vegetables that you use. The success of this diet also greatly hinges on the quality of the dairy you use. The higher the quality the dairy products, the higher chance you have of success.

# Daily Food Intake

2–4 cups of raw, whole-fat dairy per day in the form of milk, kefir, whey, yogurt, clabber, or buttermilk. You can substitute about two ounces of cheese for every cup of dairy. Also consider an eggnog smoothie as described in the next chapter.

2–4 ounces of raw cheese

1–4 eggs per day, either raw, soft-boiled or fully cooked

Plenty of vegetables such as provided by the Ayurvedic Green Drink (recipe provided in the next chapter), or vegetable soup.

Vitamin C-rich foods such as broccoli, cauliflower, bell peppers, mustard greens, cabbage, sauerkraut, kohlrabi, liver and adrenal glands.

Plenty of butter or ghee with every meal.

At least once per day have something fermented such as kefir, yogurt or sauerkraut.

Optional: Seaweed

You will want to focus on having concentrated vegetable sources as your dietary base. This is best obtained from vegetable soups or the Ayurvedic green drink discussed in the next chapter. Vegetable minerals can also be obtained from vegetable juicing if you are aware of the principles of avoiding plant toxins from juicing. As with the other dietary programs you will want to have some form of protein with every meal. Cheese is particularly concentrated in the important minerals calcium and phosphorous and is a very high quality protein. Yogurt makes a great addition to meals. Make sure to get genuine grass-fed cheese whenever possible. Be extremely careful with your use of grains in this diet. They must be phytate free. If you consume brown rice it must first be soaked with a starter as described in the next chapter, and very well cooked until the grains burst open. *If the vegetarian plan fails for you consider adding some fermented cod liver oil to the diet to provide the missing vitamins needed for success.*

## Self Care

Healing your teeth is all about taking care of yourself. In natural eco-systems undisturbed by humans it is easy to see how Nature provides for all of her creations. Plants and animals generally have plenty of food and nutrients, and they do not suffer from relentless stress. Even though we are also a part of Nature, the design and structure of our civilization is built upon the belief systems of deprivation, competition for resources, and exploitation rather than upon a belief in abundance for all. Rather than giving, our society takes, and then takes some more. The designs of our buildings and transportation systems take tremendous amounts of resources to build and maintain. The government takes our money as taxes and we can question how much of that money is being used to nurture and support citizens and social networks.

All of this taking is disharmonious, stressful and destructive. The society and world many of us live in makes it hard for us to relax. If we can relax, however, we find it is much easier to take care of ourselves. Taking care of oneself is in alignment with the law of personal responsibility. If you feel unimportant, undeserving, or unhappy, it will be difficult to take good care of yourself and give your body the food that it needs. When you truly are willing and able to take care yourself you will find healing. Allow yourself space to make your needs important and take excellent care of yourself.

## *Common Mistakes Made By People Who Think They Are Eating a Healthy Diet*

Making mistakes in food choices is very much tied to your level of self care. When you rush too much, or are unwilling or unable to take proper care of yourself, then you cut corners on food selection and health problems can result. If you think you are eating in a healthy fashion but are suffering from tooth decay, I want to remind you of some common mistakes that people often make so that you can avoid them.

> **Poor food quality**—Watch out for packaged food, even organically labeled food, as it may not be good for you. If you are a great fan of dairy products, be aware that grain-fed dairy products, even if they are raw, can cause imbalances in some people. Get the best and freshest food you are able to find.

**Skipping fat-soluble vitamins**—I have been absolutely clear on insisting that fat-soluble vitamins are of utmost importance in order to have strong teeth. If you skip this step, tooth remineralization will be difficult to achieve.

**Too much sweet food**—A sweet is a sweet. If you have cavities you must be disciplined and limit your sweets. Your teeth are worth it. Natural sweets are safer than highly refined ones, but that does not mean you can eat as much as you want and not suffer the consequences.

**Lack of minerals**—Bone broth aids in nutrient absorption and is rich in minerals. Seaweed, fish and shellfish are very rich in minerals. If you exclusively eat land animals for proteins, and they are not of a very high quality, it is possible to run into problems from nutrient deficiencies. Make sure to get high quality animal foods as farm fresh as possible. In addition, eating some of the animal organs will help fill in the missing mineral gaps.

**Poor food absorption**—Perhaps you are not digesting your food well. Focus on adding fermented foods, bone broth, kefir, raw eggs, and probiotics to aid in digestion. Consider getting support from a natural health care practitioner to help you with herbs to strengthen your digestive abilities, particularly to clean and strengthen your liver.

# *Cleansing and Fasting*

While on the topic of food, we must discuss fasting. Cleanses can be helpful, but cleanses that involve ingesting maple syrup or other excess amounts of sweets like fruit juice are not good for your teeth. If your teeth are healthy then you will be fine on a short fast. I have talked with many people who tried to cleanse or fast and their teeth have gotten worse. However for some people a very short fast of one day or less has helped. I encourage gentle cleansing, which can be done with herbs, restricted diets, raw eggs and vegetable juices. Watch out for cleansing or fasting if you are already very thin or feel hungry often.

## Heal Your Teeth in Six Weeks or Less

Controlling tooth decay means that the decay ceases to progress and that new dentin forms. Dr. Price believed that "well over 95 percent" of dental caries could be controlled with a painstakingly careful nutritional protocol. Like a broken bone, your carious teeth will get strong and mend themselves. If a tooth has a hole, pit or previous filling then that hole or pit will be strong and resilient, but it will not likely fill in.

Each time you take a bite of food, your body decides to mineralize or demineralize your teeth and bones. 24–48 hours of following the balanced protocol, provided you have increased your fat-soluble vitamin intake, should lead to a perceivable tooth remineralization. For example, you would feel less tooth sensitivity, or your teeth would feel stronger. At the beginning of the nutritional protocol used on school children, Dr. Price found that the chemical analysis of the saliva of the children showed active tooth decay. In a period of six weeks, this same analysis showed that tooth decay had stopped. Over a period of five months on the special diet, the status of the saliva continued to improve.[205] You can infer from these statistics that noticeable results should be seen in about six weeks. You can also see that damaged teeth continue to heal long after this initial six-week phase of healing. A badly damaged tooth could take months to mend itself. The good news is that you can heal your teeth with diet, and getting results starts with your next meal.

*Chapter 6*

# Stop Cavities
# with Your Next Meal
# Recipes and Meal Plans

**Eating healthy is about getting in touch with your roots.** Eating healthy is about what connects you to life. It is about what connects you to the Earth and to a feeling of being well here. One way to connect to your roots is to recall some experience of real food in your life, particularly from your past. See what comes to mind for you right now. One example might be the memory of a family member who cooked a traditional dish from your cultural heritage. Or for someone who has immigrated to the United States, it would be the favorite foods from the past from your home country that were real foods. Meals made from foods from your family's roots evoke memories of feeling connected. Often these homemade meals consisted of nutrient-dense dishes made with bone broths, organ meats, and high quality fats. From my past it was as simple as my cousins who ate wild salmon every day, and my father who would prepare a simple dinner of rice, vegetables and fish or chicken. My grandmother would make chicken soup with the entire chicken, and eat the marrow in the bones. In my more ancient roots, before I was born, my grandfather grew up where people carried animal skin bags of fresh pastured goat milk and drank from them all day. No matter where you are from, one key to finding a healthy diet for you is to go back to your own past. Maybe that connection was a special restaurant or a memorable meal in a friend's or relative's home. See if you can recall that wholesome good food from your past. Many people have grandparents who used to eat wholesome foods, or own nearly forgotten cookery books full of golden recipes for real foods. And here lies the untapped wisdom of the older generations. No matter where you live, connecting to your roots can connect you with a diet that is nourishing, life sustaining, and rich in fat-soluble vitamins. No matter where you are from, or where you live, reach for that distant but ever-so-close connection to wholesome foods. And then make it present here and now in your life. Seek out the old family recipes, contact relatives who live in far off lands, or create your own traditional foods with a little help from recipe books. It will probably take some work, but the rewards will be more health and happiness.

In this chapter I will present you with specific recipes, meal ideas and I will tackle the complex question of how to prepare grains safely.

# *Tooth Decay Healing Diets that Worked*

Doctor J.D. Boyd created a grain-free diet that turned soft cavities into hard glassy surfaces. The diet contained milk, cream, butter, eggs, meat, cod liver oil, bulky vegetables and fruit. The daily menu included one quart of milk with plenty of cream. Dietary fat came from cream, butter and egg yolks. The diet contained no processed sugar, bread or grains of any sort.

I am using a grain-free diet as the baseline of my recommendations because I want to give you material that I am certain will work. One method that I suggest for some people is to start with a low grain or grain-free diet, try it out a few weeks and then add grains gradually later so you can feel how grains affect your body.

Here is a modified outline of Dr. May Mellanby's tooth decay remineralizing diet. Each category contains several meal ideas. In this diet cod liver oil was given daily to the children and is a key element in allowing this diet to arrest cavities.

### Breakfasts

Omelet, cocoa with milk.

Scrambled egg, milk, fresh salad.

Omelet containing two ounces of ground beef.

Fish cakes with potatoes dipped in egg and fried.

Bacon, fried or finely chopped with parsley and scrambled egg.

Eggs that are boiled, fried or poached.

Fish fried or steamed.

**Lunches**—Lunch is the biggest meal of the day.

Potatoes, steamed ground beef, carrots, stewed fruit.

Irish stew (a lamb or mutton stew with soup bones), potatoes, cooked fruit and milk.

Cold meat cut into small pieces with cold diced cooked carrot, onion and potato, and served on lettuce leaf.

**Desserts**—Dessert is served after lunch rather than after dinner. This is the ideal time to have something sweet in the day.

Fresh fruit salad with egg custard or cream.

Baked apple with center filled with golden syrup before baking.

Fresh fruit salad, cocoa made with milk.

Baked apple, centre filled with maple syrup before cooking.

Honeycomb which contains bee larvae.

**Dinners or Snacks**

Minced beef warmed with meat juice and a green salad.

Potato cakes or fish cakes.

Eggs, cooked in various ways.

Fish and potatoes fried in lard or tallow with milk to drink.

Thick potato soup made with milk.

Lentil or celery soup made with milk and chopped meat.

Cheese, served in various ways.

Milk

Potatoes, steamed minced meat, carrots, cooked fruit, milk.

In Dr. Mellanby's plan lunch is the main meal of the day, and sweets are eaten after lunch not after dinner.

## Cure Tooth Decay Meal Ideas

Here is a list of tasty and nutrient-dense meal ideas. You can use these meals for breakfast, lunch, or dinner. This is by no means a complete menu, merely suggestions to work with. Ideally you will have a mixture of both sea foods and land foods. However, I understand that many people do not have access to both, or have a preference for one.

## Examples of Dishes from the Sea

**Sushi:** *Miso soup made with fish broth, seaweed and bok choy or misome.*

*Sushi rolls made with raw tuna, carrot, cucumber, avocado or sushi with smoked salmon and cream cheese.*

**Ceviche fish** *with a cup of miso soup made with fish broth.*

**Sashimi raw tuna salad** *(also known as poke) with a side of miso soup made from fish stock, with greens and/ or seaweed.*

**Lobster, clam, or oyster chowder**

**Fish cakes** *made with potatoes dipped in egg and fried in animal fat. A cup of fish broth on the side.*

**Fish sticks** *white fish, cut into long strips, homemade sourdough breadcrumbs, 2 raw eggs mixed and seasoned with sea salt and pepper, and ghee for frying. Dredge fish in egg mixture, then breadcrumbs, then fry in ghee. Make tartar sauce for the side and have with fish soup.*

**Fish head soup**

**Cioppino.** *Seafood stew, including fish stock, fish, squid, mussels, and clams.*

## Examples of Dishes from the Land

**Meat loaf** *made with 25% ground organ meats, cooked in beef stock.*

**Beef meatballs** *in beef broth marinara sauce that includes vegetables with cheese on the top. You can also add spaghetti squash and have the meat balls with vegetable spaghetti.*

**Butternut squash soup** *made with beef broth and the cream juiced from fresh coconuts (you can use coconut cream in jars as a replacement).*

**Liver with caramelized onions,** *or roasted bone marrow on sourdough bread.*

**Steak tartare** *with raw ground beef mixed with Italian herbs and mustard (for one pound ground beef, use two teaspoons of herbs and one teaspoon of mustard, and two teaspoons of finely chopped red onion, sea salt to taste. Sauerkraut and raw liver cut into small chunks on the side.*

**Kabobs.** *Shrimp, chicken pieces, lamb pieces, with liver, heart and/or kidney, assorted vegetables (peppers, zucchini, mushrooms) tossed in oil, sea salt, pepper, placed on skewers and then grilled. Side of beef broth, and corn on the cob.*

**Hamburger** *with shredded kidney fat and yam chips fried in lard or ghee on the side.*

## Examples of Side Dishes / Snacks / Other Meals

Vegetable soup

Tooth-strengthening eggnog smoothie

Pickled beets

Sauerkraut / kimchi /pickles

Omelet with mushrooms and cheese

Poi: soured sweet potatoes or taro root

Raw cheese custard with fruit *1 cup of fresh raw milk curd (the milk solids after the whey is separated) blended with 2 raw eggs, 1 teaspoon of raw honey*

Soft-boiled eggs with a dash of salt

Cheese and apples or pears

Dosas soured overnight with yogurt

Cheese and roasted nuts

One cup of raw milk

Seaweed snacks such as dried sea palm

Boiled beef tongue with minced garlic or creamed horseradish

Sweetbreads breaded with flour (nut powder or sourdough bread crumbs) and fried in lard, ghee or tallow

**Seared sweet potatoes:** *roasted sweet potatoes, sliced thickly, then pan fried in ghee, or lard.*

**Squash "cupcakes":** *roasted acorn and butternut squashes, flesh removed from peel and seeds, mashed and blended with a touch of maple syrup. Place into cupcake wrappers, and garnish with coconut cream or fresh, unsweetened raw whipped cream.*

**Stir-fried kale** *(can also be used for bok choy) chopped greens sautéed with butter, ginger, garlic, and tamari.*

**Chicken with liver.** *Fried liver with ghee (clarified butter) or lard, mushrooms and onions. Have with a side of chicken soup (soup cooked with chicken feet and heads).*

**Deviled eggs.** *Hard boiled eggs, peeled and cut in half lengthwise. Remove the yolks, mash with homemade mayonnaise, fresh chopped chives, sea salt, fresh cracked pepper, dash of mustard powder. Fill eggs with egg yolk filling.*

**Flavorful scrambled eggs.** *Include chopped onion, chopped tomato, sautéed in ghee with a dash of red cayenne pepper and a dash of turmeric.*

**Eggs Benedict on sourdough rye**—*just two fried eggs on a split sourdough rye bagel with hollandaise sauce (clarified butter with 2 raw egg yolks, dash of cayenne and lemon juice whipped until fluffy) poured over eggs.*

The menus that follow are creative concepts. These exact food combinations or having those specific meals in the same day may not work for you. Do not force yourself to eat anything, rather look for and eat the amount of food that feels good and satisfying to you.

## Sea Food Sample Menu

### Day 1

**Breakfast:** Scrambled eggs with fish eggs, sweet potatoes fried in ghee, a cup of milk. *Fermented skate or cod liver oil with butter oil.*

**Lunch:** Smoked salmon with kale that was simmered in water. Side of liver with onions.

**Snack:** Peaches in raw milk yogurt.

**Dinner:** Miso soup made with fish broth. Sushi rolls with tuna (can be raw or cooked), avocado, carrots, rice and cucumbers with wasabi and pickled ginger. *Fermented skate or cod liver oil with butter oil.*

### Day 2

**Breakfast:** Scrambled eggs with grated cheese and boiled and mashed sweet potatoes. Glass of raw milk. *Fermented skate or cod liver oil with butter oil.*

**Snack:** Blackberries with cottage cheese.

**Lunch:** Fish head soup.

**Dinner:** Vegetable soup with string beans and zucchini. Side of potatoes and rice. Chicken, fish, or sausage. *Fermented skate or cod liver oil with butter oil.*

## Land Food Sample Menu

### Day 1

**Breakfast:** Butternut squash soup made with beef broth and the cream juiced from fresh coconuts. *Fermented skate or cod liver oil with butter oil.*

**Lunch:** Hamburger with caramelized onions and mushrooms. Fermented ketchup, pickles, sauerkraut and mustard on the side in a lettuce bun. Raw liver or liver with onions on the side. Hamburger is mixed with kidney fat or cooked in tallow when available.

**Snack** —Fruit with raw milk custard made with 1 cup raw milk curds, 2 raw eggs blended with about one teaspoon of raw honey.

**Dinner** —Meatballs cooked with homemade tomato sauce made with tomato paste and beef stock. This goes great on spaghetti squash or with other squash. Plenty of cheese on top. Liver and onions on the side. *Fermented skate or cod liver oil with butter oil.*

*Day 2*

**Breakfast**—Soft cooked or scrambled eggs with goat cheese and organic baby spinach (liver, kidney, or some organ meat is needed on the side).

**Lunch**—Steak tartare with raw beef mixed with finely chopped red onion, Italian herbs, sea salt, and mustard. Sauerkraut and raw liver cut into small chunks on the side.

**Snack**—Homemade vanilla raw milk ice cream lightly sweetened with maple syrup and/ or a banana. We use about one or two tablespoons of maple syrup per quart of ice cream. Or one or two teaspoons of maple syrup with a mashed banana with the milk and cream and vanilla extract.

**Dinner**—Shish kebabs with a cup of broth on the side, and corn on the cob. Pound the steak or chicken pieces flat and marinate in teriyaki sauce over night. *Fermented skate or cod liver oil with butter oil.*

# Recipes for Healing Your Teeth

## Bone Broth Recipe

Just as a reminder, bone broths are very effective towards improving your health and encouraging tooth mineralization and should be included in your diet on a daily basis.

1. Bones—from chicken, fish, shellfish, beef, lamb

   Regular bones are fine. But ideally for chicken use chicken feet and heads. For beef and lamb knuckle bones work very well. For fish having the head with the carcass is ideal.

2. Cover the bones with water

3. Add two tablespoons of vinegar (any type) per quart of water

4. Vegetables such as carrots and onions can be added to soup stock

Making broth is not difficult. Put the bones in a pot, add water and vinegar to cover by a couple of inches and let it stand for 30–60 minutes. Bring the pot to a boil and then reduce heat to a simmer. Remove any scum at the top of the broth with a spoon. Ideally simmer for 24–48 hours. As little as 6 hours will do. Strain the broth to remove the bones. The meat on the bones or marrow inside the bones is edible.

# Bieler's Soup

This is the original healing soup of Dr. Henry Bieler, which will help strengthen your glands and provide balance to a diet rich in animal foods.

    1 pound of string beans, ends removed

    2 pounds zucchini, chopped

    1 handful of curly parsley*

    Enough water to cover your veggies

Add all ingredients to rapidly boiling water and boil for 10–15 minutes, or until a fork easily pierces the zucchini skin. Purée using the cooking water (it is important to use this water as it contains vitamins and minerals) and make the soup to the consistency you desire.

This specific recipe is designed for healing when the body is ill. Feel free to modify this recipe by adding all kinds of different vegetables to make a soup to suit your personal needs.

*Pregnant and lactating women should limit their parsley intake as it dries up breast milk.

# Eggnog Tooth-Strengthening Formula

For those who have difficulty absorbing nutrients from foods, organic or high-quality raw eggs will help heal this problem. The raw egg formula gave me food to eat when I was having difficulties digesting other types of foods. Combining raw eggs with raw milk ensures the maximum level of assimilation of nutrients from the raw milk. This mixture regenerates intestinal mucosa and helps heal leaky gut syndrome.

**Try the following blend:**

    1 cup raw milk, kefir or yogurt

    1-2 raw eggs

    optional ingredients include:

    2 ounces of raw cream

    ½ teaspoon raw honey, or organic maple syrup

    dash of nutmeg and cinnamon for flavor

    a drop or two of vanilla extract

carob or chocolate powder

To enhance assimilation, have ingredients at room temperature.

Note: If you are pregnant and eating raw eggs, then for every five days of eating raw eggs, abstain for two days.[206]

**A word of warning.** You may initially feel worse after eating raw eggs if you do not regularly eat them. Raw eggs can induce intense detoxification symptoms as your body cleanses. For example, on one occasion I ate raw farm-fresh eggs, and my body started to release and detoxify residues of Valium (a drug I had taken 15 years earlier for pain). I knew it was Valium because of its unmistakable feelings of nausea and disassociation, and I was violently ill for about one day as my body dumped the drug residues into my stomach. Afterward I ate the same eggs both raw and cooked without aversion or health problems.

**Egg whites:** Some people believe in only eating the egg whites. Others believe in eating only or mostly the egg yolks, and limiting their egg white intake because of the risk of possibly inducing a biotin deficiency. Eating only the yolk is an acceptable practice. My personal preference is to eat the whole egg.

## Spicy Steak Tartare for Fighting Tooth Infections

This raw meat recipe was used to successfully heal a tooth infection.

1 pound raw ground pastured bison, beef, or lamb

4 oz. of yellow butter

1 teaspoon of cayenne pepper or fresh spicy chilies

1 tablespoon of raw, unheated honey

Place butter, cayenne, and raw honey in a glass jar or bowl. Then immerse that bowl in a bowl of hot water that is not too hot. A double boiler turned on low will suffice. You must not raise the temperature of the food above 93 degrees Fahrenheit in order to preserve the enzymes. Once the butter/honey/cayenne mixture is melted, add the ground bison and stir. This is a healthy raw food dish.

If you try this recipe with cooked meat, your success rate will be greatly diminished.

Cayenne pepper is used in many natural healing remedies and can promote the healing of tooth infections.

## Fish Head Soup

Fish head soup is a delicacy in many parts of the world. The basic concept of fish head soup is boiled fish heads and flavoring. This soup will be richer if prepared with fish stock, but it can also be prepared with water only. I chose a recipe here that does not retain the whole fish head, but when the head is floating in the soup it is much more fun.

½ to 2 pounds of fish heads. Remove the gills before making the soup and clean head thoroughly with water. Fill your soup pot with water just up to the heads or slightly below.

Simmer with 1–2 tablespoons of thinly sliced ginger for 15–30 minutes.

Strain the broth.

Pick all of the meat and soft tissues off the bones. Anything that is soft is edible. Return the meat to the broth.

There are many variations of the soup. You can sauté any or all of the following with sesame oil, fish sauce or wine including onions, garlic, leeks, bamboo shoots, and red peppers. You can also add cabbage or other vegetables while the soup is cooking. Alternatively make a creamy soup with cream and potatoes like a fish head chowder.

## Ayurvedic Green Drink

Many ancient traditions including Ayurveda believe that most vegetables need to be eaten cooked, not raw. This recipe provides the green goodness of vegetables with spices and calcium to provide a nutrient rich-smoothie or soup.

¼ teaspoon natural salt

¼ teaspoon turmeric

1 teaspoon garam masala

1 tablespoon of ghee

8 ounces of water

16 ounces of fresh vegetables

4 ounces of paneer raw or cooked (cheese curd)

1. Make paneer.

2. Add turmeric, salt, water, oil, and cook for 15 minutes.

3. Add greens and masala and cover with glass top. Watch for brightness in the green color of the vegetables. When you see a rich brilliant green, stop cooking. Blend the vegetables with the paneer and serve with lime.

**Cooked Paneer**

4 cups whole fresh milk

3-4 teaspoons of natural acid from fresh lime juice, lemon juice, or vinegar.

1. Heat milk to just below boiling, stir often while heating. When the milk is just below boiling turn off the heat.

2. Add acidic substance one teaspoon at a time while stirring. When you add the correct amount it will immediately curdle.

3. Strain with cheese cloth or clean towel to separate curds from whey.

4. Wrap curds in cloth and let it hang over a pot or bowl for one hour to remove the remaining liquid. The curds are paneer. You can further refrigerate and press it into little cheese blocks. You can use the whey for a drink by mixing it with lime or orange juice, or you can also add it to soups as a base.

**Raw Paneer**

If you want to use a raw dairy product with this smoothie, then you will want to sour milk by leaving it out in a glass jar for several days until the whey separates. Strain out the whey with a cloth. The solids of the soured milk can substitute as a paneer replacement but it won't be as firm.

# Poke (pronounced POH-kay) Fish Salad

1 pound fresh or sashimi-grade tuna, cut into small cubes

2–3 stalks of green onion chopped

½ cup soy sauce

2 tablespoons sesame seed oil

1 tablespoon grated fresh ginger

Splash of vinegar and salt and pepper to taste

**Optional variations**: 2 tablespoons olive oil, chili peppers finely minced, toasted sesame seeds, small pieces of celery, chunks of avocado, cucumber

In a large bowl, combine tuna, soy sauce, green onions, sesame oil, ginger, salt, and mix lightly. Cover and refrigerate two hours or more before serving to let the flavors blend. This can be served on a bed of lettuce.

# Cooking Suggestions

I do not recommend using a microwave for cooking. Microwave ovens are the only cooking source that needs a shield. Yes, regular ovens have a heat shield, but you can still open them when they are operating and you will be fine. Studies show that microwaved food can pose a greater health risk than foods cooked by other conventional means.[207] Also watch out for aluminum cookware. At home we use cast iron and high quality stainless steel cooking vessels. Other methods of cooking to retain flavor of the foods include clay pots and copper pots lined with tin. The copper pots are very expensive and if the tin coating is scraped and the copper is exposed to the food it can be toxic to use.

# Preparing Grains So That They Do Not Cause Cavities or Disease

The presence of lectins, phytic acid and other anti-nutrients in grains and beans means that they need to be carefully prepared in order to prevent them from causing tooth decay. My disclaimer on these conventions is that I cannot tell you for certain that these methods will not cause cavities. By reviewing indigenous cultures' grain preparation techniques in chapter four, you can see that part of healthy grain preparation is using specific varieties of grains, fresh grinding, aging, sifting and sun drying the grains. It is difficult to replicate every step of the process. How safe grains are to consume also depends on your level of health and ability to digest grains.

How much effort is required to prepare whole grains to make them healthy to consume depends on how much you eat. The more grains or beans you eat, the more careful you need to be with the preparation methods.

There is an upper limit to how much phytic acid we can have in our diet without producing negative effects to our teeth and bones regardless of how much vitamin A and D our diets provide. To make grains healthy to eat, we want to remove as much as we can of phytic acid and lectins.

## Phytase Content of Grains

Phytase is the enzyme needed to transform phytic acid into phosphorous through the fermentation process. In order to sour or ferment your grains to remove phytic acid, there needs to be substantial amounts of phytase. Grains are listed by the concentration of phytase. Rye, wheat, buckwheat, barley all have fairly high amounts of phytase. Amaranth and quinoa have moderate amounts. Mung beans, lentils, millet, peas, rice, corn, sorghum and oats are all very low in phytase and they do not have enough phytase in them to disable phytic acid from soaking or souring without a starter. Three days of sprouting in laboratory conditions increases phytase respectably for mung beans, lentils, millet, and corn.[208]

## *Phytic Acid Removal Summary*

To remove phytic acid you need warmth, moisture, the enzyme phytase, and the absence of too much calcium. Adding the equivalent amount of calcium contained in about two tablespoons of yogurt (40mg of calcium) to ¾ cup of flour reduced the amount of phytic acid dissolved by 50%.[209]

Without going into the details of the specific figures, it is important to understand that all whole grains, nuts, seeds and beans contain substantial amounts of phytic acid. There are no commonly available low-phytic acid whole grains. Therefore I do not recommend any shortcuts for whole grain preparation.

# Vibrant Sourdough

You will need to use your own sourdough recipe for reference. I believe the best sourdough would be produced by sprouting rye for 2–3 days and then drying it. Fresh grind the dry rye grains. Sift out 25% of the mixture removing a large portion of the heavy particles. Knead the dough very well and sour for at least 16 hours at 75 degrees F or warmer.

# Oat Preparation

I do not want to endorse oat consumption because I do not know all the requirements for certain for safe oat consumption. If you want to eat oats, here is how to remove the phytic acid. Start with raw oats. Germinating oats for 5 days at 11 degrees C (52 F) and incubation (souring) for 17 hours at (120 F) removed 98% of phytates. Alternatively sprout the oats, crush them and then sour them for two days. Soaking, germinating and souring oats with a starter will remove phytic acid. The problem is that most store-bought oats are heat treated and cannot be germinated.

# *Quinoa Preparation and Phytic Acid Removal*

Cooked for 25 minutes at 212 degrees F removes 15–20 percent of phytic acid.

Soaked for 12–14 hours at 68 degrees F, then cooked removes 60–77 percent of phytic acid.

Fermented with whey 16–18 hours at 86 degrees F, then cooked removes 82-88 percent phytic acid.

Soaked 12–14 hours, germinated 30 hours, lacto-fermented 16–18 hours, then cooked at 212 degrees F for 25 minutes removes 97–98 percent of phytic acid.

## *Preparing Brown Rice without Phytic Acid*

If you eat brown rice with any regularity I recommend removing the phytic acid through this method. Since brown rice is low in the enzyme phytase, a starter is used to increase the enzyme content and break down the phytic acid. Brown rice needs to be thoroughly cooked until the rice burst open. Even better than whole brown rice is cooking with a partially milled rice in which some of the bran is removed. Alter Eco™ Fair Trade sells semi-polished red rice. Ethnic food stores may also carry this type of rice.

1. Soak brown rice in clean water for 16–24 hours at room temperature, without changing the water. Reserve 10 percent of the soaking liquid (which should keep for a long time in the fridge). Discard remaining soaking liquid. Cook rice with clean water. This will break down about 30–50 percent of the phytic acid.

2. The next time you make brown rice, use the same procedure as above with a fresh batch of clean water, and add the 10 percent soaking liquid reserved from the last batch. This will break down more phytic acid.

3. Repeat the cycle of fresh water soaking with the previous 10 percent reserve. The process will gradually improve until 96 percent or more of the phytic acid is degraded at 24 hours. It takes about four rounds to get to 96 percent.[210]

Note: You can prepare a phytase-rich starter using small batches of brown rice in case you don't want to eat the higher phytate rice.

In the ancient Vedic diet, rice would always be prepared with turmeric, cardamom, cinnamon, cloves and other pungent spices which have a synergistic effect against rice anti-nutrients as well as enhance overall digestion.

*Chapter 7*

# Healthy Gums Lead to Healthy Teeth

**Having healthy gums will significantly aid** your chances of having healthy teeth. Healthy gums also will improve your overall health and resistance to disease. Gum disease has been directly correlated as a significant risk factor for heart disease and stroke.[211] Most people are not even aware that they have the beginnings of gum disease. Symptoms of gum disease include receding, swollen and bleeding gums, loose teeth, increased gum pocket size, dying gum tissue and tooth loss. Periodontal disease, pyorrhea, and gingivitis are some of the many names for different types and stages of gum disease. About 75% of the US population is afflicted with gum disease. As with tooth decay, gum disease gets worse with age.[212] This is not because gum disease is a part of the aging process, but it is a symptom of physical decay and degeneration that results from our modern lifestyle.

Dentist W.D. Miller, the originator of the most commonly held theory of the etiology of tooth decay, believed that one of the essential keys to immunity to tooth decay was "the protection of the neck of the tooth by healthy gums." Even if you do not have any noticeable gum disease, the advice in this chapter will teach you how to make your gums healthier. And healthier gums mean healthier teeth and a healthier body.

I am going to share with you the best of the best solutions that have rapidly induced healing in gum tissues. There is no guarantee that these methods will work for you. And not all of this advice may be suitable or accurate for someone with severe gum disease and concurrent loss of teeth.

Gum disease is a disease of modern humans. Weston Price explains:

> *Many primitive peoples not only retain all of their teeth, many of them to an old age, but also have a healthy flesh supporting these teeth. This has occurred in spite of the fact that the primitives have not had dentists to remove the deposits and no means for doing so for themselves.*[213]

Many ancient skulls found around the planet still have most or all of their teeth firmly rooted. So tooth loss from gum disease was either rare or non-existent in our ancestors.

## Dental Plaque and Gum Disease

Plaque occurs when your body chemistry is out of balance. The plaque I am referring to is the buildup of debris that sticks to your teeth in an unhealthy way. Particularly, cooked animal proteins that are not fully digested seem to cause dental plaque.

Calculus deposits are caused by a high level of blood calcium.[214] The calcium level in your bloodstream has to do with the type of calcium food sources you eat, as well as your body's ability to metabolize the calcium. Calculus appears when there is an excess of calcium in the blood compared to the amount of phosphorus in the blood.[215] Increased calculus deposits can be caused when the form of calcium in your diet is not absorbable. Nonabsorbable calcium creates free calcium in your bloodstream.

What this means is that plaque is not the root cause of gum disease. Rather plaque appears on the teeth when the body's internal chemistry is out of synchronization. This is caused by a faulty diet, excess sugar, incorrectly prepared whole grains and environmental stresses and toxins.

## Gum Disease, Bleeding, Swollen Gums and Fat-Soluble Vitamins

Pyorrhea is an advanced stage of gum disease in which ligaments and bones that support the teeth become inflamed and infected. It is partially a result of the process whereby important nutrients are not deposited into the gums because they are missing from the diet. When our body chemistry is out of balance through the over consumption of sweet and processed foods, or the under consumption of minerals, or a build-up of toxic material in the body, gum disease can result. Dr. Price explained:

> Much of what we have thought of as so-called pyorrhea in which the bone is progressively lost from around the teeth, thus allowing them to loosen, constitutes one of the most common phases of the borrowing process. This tissue with its lowered defense rapidly becomes infected and we think of the process largely in terms of that infection. A part of the local process includes the deposit of so-called calculus and tartar about the teeth. These contain toxic substances which greatly irritate the flesh, starting an inflammatory reaction. Pyorrhea in the light of our newer knowledge is largely a nutritional problem.[216]

According to Dr. Page, a calcium deficiency or excess phosphorus in the blood is the more specific cause of gum disease.

*Pyorrhea, an inflamed condition of the gums, generally occurs when the glands are malfunctioning, causing a high phosphorus level. By reducing the phosphorus to its proper relation to calcium, inflammation can be eliminated.*

When the phosphorus level of the blood is too high in proportion to calcium, there will be free phosphorus in the blood which can cause both the presence of calculus and irritated gums. When the phosphorus level was reduced to be in balance with the level of calcium in the blood the irritation (gingivitis) usually cleared up.[217] Fat-soluble vitamin D has the effect of lowering blood phosphorous and raising blood calcium. Vitamin D deficiency is responsible for problems with the hard areas under the gums such as the alveolar bone which comprises the tooth socket.[218]

Interestingly enough, Dr. Mellanby in his dog experiments found that fat-soluble vitamin A controlled the process and development of gum tissues. If young dogs are fed diets deficient in vitamin A, gum tissues can become swollen and overgrown. Once the gum tissue is swollen, microorganisms can be found present.[219] Vitamin A stimulates certain growth factors and perhaps this explains vitamin A's effect on gum tissues.

A key strategy in your treatment of gum disease is to use both fat-soluble vitamin A for the soft tissues and fat-soluble vitamin D for the harder tissues and bone. If you are leaning to the idea that fat-soluble vitamin A is more important, then I would recommend eating liver.

Gum disease is also connected with an overactive anterior pituitary gland. One of the roles of the anterior pituitary gland is to produce growth hormones; this gland is balanced with testosterone or estrogen. The lack of growth hormone production is therefore intimately connected with gum disease. Testosterone or estrogen can be increased by moderate exercise, making sure your weight is in your ideal range, a variety of herbal remedies, and avoiding alcohol.

## Gum Disease, Vitamin C, and Scurvy

Guinea pigs kept on a vitamin C-deficient diet which produces scurvy eventually show signs of gum disease. Their teeth become elongated from the receding gums which become red and spongy. On the same hand, successful reports of healing gum disease involve vitamin C supplementation such as with camu camu berry. Other foods highly concentrated in vitamin C are amalaki berry, acerola cherry and rose hips. Take as much as two teaspoons of powdered vitamin C-rich berries per day. Synthetic vitamin C in the form of ascorbic acid may still be effective in healing gum disease, but it is unclear as to how effective it will be. Two teaspoons of vitamin C-rich berries provides about 225 milligrams of vitamin C. For maintenance of gum health a much smaller dose should work. It is also possible that a much smaller dose of natural vitamin C will work if there are not too many whole grains in your diet.

An early treatment for infantile scurvy was raw milk and raw meat. Both foods contain highly digestible forms of phosphorous. These foods will also help heal gum disease. You do not have to eat raw meat. Another option is meat cooked in bone broth stews.

# The Amazing Blotting Technique and Healing Gum Disease Naturally

Forget about expensive gum disease surgery. The late dentist Joseph Phillips discovered a highly effective treatment method for gum disease. He also has some remarkable comments on the causes of gum disease. Instead of believing that gum disease results from buildup of tartar, Dr. Phillips was convinced it was the other way around: tartar is actually the result of gum disease.[220] Dr. Phillips went as far as stating that, "The truth of the matter is that brushing and flossing causes periodontal disease." As time goes on, Dr. Phillips believed that more brushing and flossing causes more gum disease. This is because the normal motion of tooth brushing concentrates the tooth tartar at the gum line where it is left to fester. The gum line area known as the gingival sulcus is always the dirtiest after brushing.[221] The irritating substances constantly contacting the gum tissues usually causes the gums to recede or become inflamed over time. When this area is not cleaned carefully after brushing with blotting, or an oral irrigator, then brushing will contribute to gum disease.

## How to Blot at Home

The blotting technique is so effective you can expect to see noticeable results within three weeks in a high proportion of cases. Part of the blotting technique is to clean all of the soft tissue surfaces in your mouth with a gum toothbrush. The complete technique is rather difficult to explain accurately in the text without showing you a video, so I have created a free online resource with a video to show you how to blot at home. If you want to learn how to blot at home, then please go to this website.

www.curetoothdecay.com/blotting

# Sea Salt for Your Gums

Dentist Robert Nara discovered that when treating gum disease in the military, rather than resort to time-consuming gum surgery, if he just had his patients brush their teeth and rinse their mouths with a sea salt solution, then their gum problems typically improved and were even cured. This work eventually led him to write *How to Become Dentally Self Sufficient.* The premise of the book is that good oral hygiene, including the use of oral irrigation and sea salt, will prevent or significantly reduce most tooth and gum problems.

The use of oral irrigating devices such as a Waterpik® is highly effective in treating gum disease. In case it is not clear, an oral irrigator is a device that shoots a pressurized stream of water out of a small nozzle that can clean around the teeth below the gum lines. Flossing does not reach these same places. Irrigators are available in most drug stores.

The most effective method for healing gum problems is to rinse your mouth with warm salt water using an oral irrigator. Sea salt or equivalent high quality salt would be ideal for this; do not use commercial table salt. Warm sea salt water used in an irrigating device is one of the best protections against gum disease. I have heard claims that sea salt in the oral irrigator may shorten its life span. This could be true, but the benefits surely outweigh the cost. Alternatively a teaspoon or two of apple cider vinegar diluted in the oral irrigator water can also help with gum health. Herbal liquids for gum disease can also be used in the oral irrigator and injected deep into inflamed gum tissues.

. . . . . . . . . . . . . . . . . . . . . . . . . . . . . . . . . . . . . . . . . . . . . . . .

**No More Bad Breath**

Bad breath is many times caused by decaying food trapped below the gum line. Oral irrigating with warm salt water or blotting will relieve or improve many cases of bad breath by removing the rotting food particles.

. . . . . . . . . . . . . . . . . . . . . . . . . . . . . . . . . . . . . . . . . . . . . . . .

Use an oral irrigator according to the instructions provided. The nozzle tip of the irrigator is pointed at the base of the tooth, and then the irrigator is run around the tooth. If there is pain or bleeding gums, decrease the pressure. As your gums heal and strengthen this should go away quickly.

The results from this process are gradual. Many people report healing of their gum tissues over a period of a few weeks to a few months. Even though it takes time, the results are very satisfying.

# *Herbal Treatments for Gum Disease*

People have written that herbal treatments have done wonders for their gum problems. These treatments may also help strengthen your teeth and the ligaments that hold the teeth in their sockets. Herbs that are excellent for healing teeth include:

**White oak bark powder**—prevents the need for gum surgery and heals bleeding and infected gums.

**Myrrh gum powder**—heals gum infections.

*Tooth and Gum Restore Formula* by Dr. Richard Schulze (this can be used with an oral irrigator).

*Herbal Tooth & Gum Powder* by Dr. Christopher (the recipe is in chapter 8).

There are many other herbs that can help heal teeth and gums that are not mentioned here. Alternative treatments like trigger point massage and acupressure can also help.

# Oil Pulling for your Teeth and Gums

Oil pulling is the simple but ancient technique of swishing oil in your mouth as a mouthwash. Use about one tablespoon of organic oil. Coconut and sesame seed oil work well, and olive oil is another option. Swish the oil around as long as you can. 10-20 minutes is ideal but it can be difficult to go that long. Spit the oil out when you are done (not in your sink) and rinse your mouth well. The oil pulls out toxins from your gum tissues and helps remove deeply embedded debris. This is a great treatment for gum problems, bad breath, or to increase your overall oral health

**Mercury and Your Gums**

A common symptom of mercury toxicity is bleeding gums and loose teeth.[222]

# Healing Gum Disease Program

Since scurvy and a vitamin C deficiency are easily caused by a diet heavy in whole grains, I recommend being extremely careful with the use of grain bran and grain germ in your healing gum disease diet. In addition to being alert to the toxic factors in whole grains, avoiding the toxic foods mentioned in the previous chapters will help fight gum disease. If any of the supplemental foods mentioned here are already in your diet, then you do not need to take them twice. When your gum disease is gone, then pick and choose aspects of this program to your liking.

1–2 teaspoons of food-based vitamin C from concentrated sources such as camu camu berry, acerola cherry, amalaki or rose hips for vitamin C. 2 teaspoons of camu camu berry provides about 225 milligrams of natural vitamin C.

¼–½ teaspoon 2-3 times per day for a teens and adults for a total of ½ – 1½ teaspoons per day Blue Ice™ fermented cod liver oil (available at **codliveroilshop.com**). This is to restore fat-soluble vitamins A and D to the diet for gum health.

Raw milk and/or raw meat (meat in stews is a second-best option).

Avoid whole grains unless freshly ground, soured, and appropriately sifted to remove the bran and germ.

Use the blotting technique and/or an oral irrigator with warm water and sea salt at least twice per day.

Practice oil pulling at least once per day.

Pick one topical herb or additional treatment to support your gum health.

Check if you have mercury poisoning from amalgam fillings and consider replacing them. (Mercury poisoning is discussed in chapter 8.)

Eat iron-containing foods as well as foods that enhance iron absorption such as beef, lamb, liver, clams or leafy green vegetables.

Avoid mouthwashes that are anti-bacterial that contain chemicals. We do not want to kill the good bacteria.

Avoid normal tooth brushing that irritates your gums.

*Chapter 8*

# Dentistry and its High Price

**Modern dentistry is a profound failure.** The enormity of suffering and disease caused by dentistry is so massive that is beyond comprehension. Dentistry is built on the false premise that bacteria cause cavities. Its treatment methods of drilling and filling are highly damaging to teeth. The materials used in dentistry are extremely toxic and have been connected to diseases that are severe, painful and widespread. Conventional dentistry has placed highly poisonous mercury in the mouths of hundreds of millions of people. The mercury exposure of dentists and suffering caused by dentistry explains in part why dentists have one of the highest suicide rates of any profession. Tens of millions of needless root canals have been performed. Modern dentistry has drilled deeply into healthy parts of millions of teeth because of the failed treatment policy of "extension for prevention." It has caused irreversible pulp damage in millions of tooth nerves with drills that spin too fast. The profit-motivated system of dentistry has led to tens of millions of needless dental procedures. Modern dentistry has poisoned tens of millions of children by promoting the topical and internal use of the unproven poison fluoride. And dentistry has in some cases killed innocent children slowly from the side effects of dental surgery, from swallowing fluoride, and from deadly side effects of disease-inciting metals implanted in children's mouths. If this dental massacre had any benefits to show then perhaps it could be exonerated. But it does not. After the age of sixty, the average individual has more than half of the teeth affected by tooth decay. And after this age, the average person has lost more than eight teeth, not including the wisdom teeth.

Many of us are literally carrying around dental trauma as mercury fillings from this war on bacteria. I myself am also a victim. I had seven mercury-based fillings placed during my teenage years. None of these teeth ever hurt me prior to their butchery by the dental drill. During a checkup large holes were drilled unnecessarily into my teeth because of some tiny specks that appeared on an x-ray. Each one of those teeth is now permanently and irrevocably damaged from the excavations of the dental drill. I will discuss the disaster of modern orthodontics in the next chapter.

In light of all this, when people are hesitant to go to the dentist, or are afraid of the dentist, I am not surprised. **How could you not be afraid of the dentist?**

In this chapter you will learn how to navigate through the swamp of bad dentistry. You will learn what the hazards of conventional dentistry are and how to avoid them. You will learn how to locate the few good dentists that are out there to help you repair all the toxic and damaging dental work from the past. You will learn how to communicate effectively with your dentist so that he serves your needs. I will help guide you in understanding and identifying what exactly is and has happened to your tooth that is causing you pain, so that you can take steps to resolve it with nutrition only, with surgery, or with both.

# Toxic Dentistry

Conventional dentists drill holes in your teeth in exchange for money and then place a poisonous substance in your mouth (mercury fillings) to prevent bacteria from making a hole in your teeth.

Conventional dentistry is so bad that many conscientious dentists are doing their best to get the word out to the public. A majority of dentists who have become holistically oriented did not even start out with a holistic mindset. Generally their transformation was inspired after a painful wakeup call, such as their own symptoms of mercury poisoning, or the dentist sees the dreaded result of their poor dental care failing their patients, or themselves. As a result, many dentists who see the problems inherent in conventional dentistry feel extreme remorse for their years in practice of toxic dentistry. And a few of the dentists who feel a duty to prevent the shameful practice of modern dentistry to continue make a good effort to inform the public about diseases caused by dentistry. Some have even written books in order to inform the public about the extreme danger that may be lurking in our mouths. These books are valuable supplemental readings to this one, especially if you want more details about the problems with dental materials and dentistry. They include *Whole Body Dentistry* by dentist Mark Breiner, published in 1999; *Uniformed Consent* by dentist Hal Huggins, published in 1999; *The Key to Ultimate Health* by Ellen Brown and dentist Richard Hansen, 1998; *It's All In Your Head: the link between mercury amalgams and illness* by Dr. Hal Huggins, 1993; *Are Your Dental Fillings Poisoning You?* by dentist Guy Fasciana, published in 1986; *Dental Infections* by Weston Price.

## Diseases and Mercury

The first reported case of Hodgkin's lymphoma was recorded in 1832 shortly after the first amalgam fillings were used. Dr. Olympio Pinto introduced the subject of mercury toxicity to Dr. Hal Huggins in 1973. When finishing his master's degree at Georgetown University Dr. Pinto's thesis topic was mercury toxicity. His thesis was never published because the National Institute of Dental Research, part of the National Institutes of Health, found out about his project and stopped it.[223] Dr. Huggins eventually published the material himself in the *Journal of the International Academy of Preventative Medicine* in 1976.

That mercury fillings are highly toxic is without question. According to the

US government's Agency for Toxic Substances and Disease Registry mercury is ranked #3 of the most toxic chemicals or metals on the planet. Arsenic and lead are slightly ahead of it, but chloroform, cyanide, and plutonium are less toxic to humans than mercury.[224] Mercury fillings are also wrongly called amalgam fillings or silver fillings to disguise their main ingredient, mercury. Mercury accounts for approximately 50% of a mercury filling. Imagine if you had a plutonium filling or a cyanide filling that this filling would probably be safer for you than a mercury filling depending on how fast those poisons released from the fillings.

A report by the Agency for Toxic Substances and Disease Registry restricts the safe level of mercury vapor for the average person to 0.28 micrograms. Various studies report that the average intake of mercury vapor from mercury amalgams is between 4-19 micrograms, in other words 10-50 times higher than the safe level of mercury vapor.[225] Studies on 10-year-old fillings show that a large portion of mercury has leaked out and evaporated by the end of the ten years. It has leaked directly into the individual's body. Unfortunately the mercury loss does not make the fillings any safer to keep in your mouth, as the mercury continually leaks out at the same rate for years and years. Due to a relatively recent lawsuit settlement, the U.S. Food and Drug Administration is now forced to admit that silver fillings containing mercury "may have neurotoxic effects on the nervous systems of developing children and fetuses."[226]

Mercury is so poisonous that it and metal dental filling materials are known to cause birth defects, chronic fatigue, indigestion, leukemia, hormonal imbalances, fibromyalgia, seizures, arthritis, Bell's palsy, allergies, and multiple sclerosis. Mercury fillings are banned in many countries including Sweden, Germany, and Japan.

Despite this evidence, and volumes more about the extreme danger of mercury in the body, the code of ethics of the American Dental Association specifically prohibits dentists from telling patients to remove their mercury fillings because mercury is toxic.

> *ADA Code of Conduct 5.A.1 Dental Amalgam and other Restorative Materials "[R]emoval of amalgam restorations... for the alleged purpose of removing toxic substances from the body, when such a treatment is performed solely at the recommendation or suggestion of the dentist, is improper and unethical."*[227]

Dentists who are caught disobeying the ADA code of conduct can lose their license. Dentists are allowed to remove mercury fillings by your request, your doctor's request, or if your fillings are damaged. But they cannot say that they advise removing functional mercury fillings because mercury is toxic. What happened to the dentist's constitutional right of free speech and the ancient oath of the physician to "first, do no harm"?

# What to Do About Current Mercury Fillings?

There is no question that mercury fillings are highly toxic. Yet many people are able to resist this toxicity for quite some time. The most concentrated exposure to mercury comes when fillings are placed and when they are removed. Healthy people have high levels of glutathione and other substances which naturally detoxify the effects of the mercury fillings. As people age or if they are in otherwise poor health, their resistance to mercury poisoning from the fillings decreases, and thus the fillings will eventually lead to disease. If you think your fillings might be making you sick, seek the advice of a mercury-free dentist, a holistic M.D., or a naturopathic doctor who can perform a mercury challenge test to see if indeed you are retaining mercury.

Replacing mercury fillings must be done with extreme care and timing. If your dentist does not follow a careful protocol that includes protective devices such as a rubber dam, vacuum for the vapors, and a mask, then you could be exposed to microscopic mercury particles and mercury fumes that are highly toxic. At least six people have contacted me complaining of relentless tooth pain after having their amalgam fillings replaced. The drill got too close to the nerve and was over stimulated. Having several teeth drilled to remove mercury fillings in someone with a sensitive system can explain this negative result. Some people whose bite is out of position will have an already hypersensitive nervous system. This hypersensitivity is compounded by dental drilling to remove mercury from several teeth and can overwhelm the nervous system.

The other problem I have encountered is people who remove their mercury fillings yet feel no difference in their health. Removing mercury fillings for most people should lead to a noticeable improvement in energy levels, or a sense of relaxation in the body. The likely reason why people did not notice any improvement from removing their mercury fillings is because it was not done correctly, and because the replacement composite may also have been toxic. Another important detail in removing mercury is the order in which the mercury fillings are removed. Each mercury filling exerts an electrical charge. Fillings create an electrical current when the five metals in the filling combine with saliva to create a battery effect. The electrical charge is much stronger than what our nervous system runs on and it can interfere with brain and heart function.[228] The charge of each filling dictates the order in which they need to be removed. When people have dramatic and noticeable results from removing mercury fillings it is from a change in electrical currents which allows the individual's nervous system to function properly.[229]

Yes, mercury fillings are highly poisonous and need to be removed carefully. But for some people the timing is not right to immediately have them replaced. Contacting an excellent dentist from the resource list provided in this chapter will help you ensure that when you remove your old fillings, it is done in a way that does not make you sicker and with the appropriate timing. Before your dental procedure you will want to take plenty of Activator X rich-butter and cod liver oil. But you will not want to take too much oral vitamin C, since vitamin C interferes with Novocain's effects. Part of the holistic mercury removal protocol is the administration of intravenous vitamin C, which acts differently from oral supplementation of vitamin C.

## Mercury Fillings Lead To Crowns and Root Canals

Mercury amalgam fillings lead to the need to have root canals and crowns. As a filling material, mercury fillings do not reinforce the strength of teeth. With the "extension for prevention" treatment philosophy sound parts of the teeth are drilled away in order to place mercury fillings in a wedge shape. Thousands of cases illustrate that teeth restored with mercury fillings are the ones that will eventually need crowns or root canals.[230] When 30% of a tooth is drilled out to place an amalgam filling, the tooth can lose up to 80% of its strength. When the mercury filling is in place, the tooth still does not regain its lost strength. Our teeth are under tremendous biting forces. When we bite on the tooth with a mercury filling, that tooth can have stress placed upon it in the wrong spots, causing cracking, or a slow crumbling around the area where the mercury filling meets the tooth. This loss of structural integrity, in combination with a poor diet that does not permit the tooth to recover from its stress, eventually causes the tooth to fracture. I have not even mentioned that the mercury leaking out of the filling will poison the bone-building cells within the tooth. Over time the mercury-laden tooth can continue to weaken, and eventually the severe damage requires an equally severe treatment to save it, such as a crown or a root canal.

## More Dental Dangers from Toxic Dentistry

### Battery Mouth

Your body and nervous system operate on a very small electrical current. Metal fillings can produce electrical currents that can be exponentially stronger than the electrical currents in your body. Considering that your teeth are connected to the largest sensory nerve in your body, the trigeminal nerve, this excess of electricity can cause harm. The mix of metals in the mouth greatly magnifies the problems of electrical current. For example gold and mercury, or crowns that are reinforced with "stainless steel," can all be present in a mouth also containing mercury fillings. Dissimilar metals in the mouth can be responsible for neurological problems including migraine headaches.

Composite fillings also interfere with the natural electrical current of the teeth. Rather than greatly magnify it, however, composites completely dampen the current since they are made from plastic and plastic does not conduct an electrical current.

## Gold Fillings and Crowns

Pure gold is naturally quite soft. This makes it a bad dental material. It needs to be mixed with other metals to make it stronger. While it is possible that not many people's immune systems would react negatively to gold by itself, the other metals in gold fillings such as palladium can pose an immune system challenge.[231] Dental gold has an affinity for mercury released from "silver" mercury amalgam fillings. The gold attracts and stores the released mercury from other fillings. Then when exposed to heat such as a hot drink, toxic mercury vapor will release from the gold crowns.[232]

To place crowns requires extra grinding down of the tooth. This is done because of the weak bonding strength of dental cement. Dentists using new bonding technologies can avoid placing crowns, or remove significantly less of the tooth to place a crown.[233]

## Nickel and Stainless Steel

Stainless steel contains nickel. Nickel is used in braces, bridges, partials and crowns. Nickel is a metal that is highly toxic the body. Nickel is hidden in crowns and metal jackets for children's tooth cavities and creates a negative electrical current in the mouth.[234] Nickel is highly toxic to the nervous system and may be related to arthritis and some types of cancer such as lung cancer and breast cancer.[235] Nickel is used to induce cancer in laboratory animals.[236]

## Porcelain as a Dental Material

Porcelain contains aluminum in the form of aluminum oxide. Aluminum is toxic to humans. The official belief in dentistry regarding the stability of aluminum in porcelain is identical to the official belief of mercury's safety in amalgam. Aluminum is purported to remain bonded to the other materials in porcelain and not leak, but this is not likely the case.[237] Porcelain crowns are often reinforced with low-cost stainless steel which often contains nickel.[238]

# Safer Filling Materials

There are at least three holistic paradigms for safe dental filling materials. I cannot determine which one is best. I suggest you choose one that feels good for you after you have done your own investigations. As important as filling materials are, what is equally or more important is the quality of the dental work. My perspective on determining filling materials is first to find a dentist with whom you feel comfortable and trust, and who abides by a biocompatible paradigm. The premise of biocompatible dentistry is that you do not place just any material in some-body's body and hope that everything will be all right. Biocompatible dentistry aims to test and confirm that the filling materials will not adversely affect your health. One sophisticated but accurate approach to test filling materials is to get a sample vial of the filling material from your dentist, and find an osteopath, or cra-nial sacral therapist who can check how your cranial / sacral rhythm is influenced by the filling material. Electro-dermal screening, blood testing and muscle testing are other methods to determine how safe filling materials are for you. Holistically oriented dentists typically either subscribe to one of the following paradigms and offer treatments accordingly, or offer many of these treatments and they decide with the patient which treatment perspective to pursue.

**Dentist Hal Huggins**—Dr. Huggins developed a careful program for remov-ing mercury fillings and placing compatible replacements. It is based on a blood chemistry test in which your blood is checked with a database of filling materials to match for immune system compatibility.

**Dentist Douglas Cook**—Dr. Cook has tested a variety of filling materials and believes that Holistore by Den-Mat for smaller fillings and Premise Indirect (formally BelleGlass) unshaded for large cavities are the best filling materi-als.[239] Slow speed drilling prevents damage to teeth during removal.

**Dr. Robert Marshall**—Electrical testing shows that composite materials block vital electrical flows to the body, while metals overly increase them and are toxic. Therefore from Dr. Marshall's perspective, the only safe dental materi-als are low-fusing ceramics laser bonded to the teeth. Low-fusing ceramics and ceramic resin hybrids allow a slight electrical current and mimic the function of natural tooth. These materials include Degussa Ceramic, Vita-block, Luminesse, Cercon, Procera Zirconium, and Esthet-X composite.[240]

The disadvantage to the low-fusing ceramics is that they can cost significantly more than other filling materials and they may in certain cases require more of the tooth to be drilled.

# Finding a Good Dentist

At a conference I talked with a dentist who really seemed to understand mini-mally invasive dentistry. When I asked if I could put him on my website referral list he declined because his practice was already too full. Another popular holistic dentist in the Los Angeles area has a three-month waiting list. The cranial dental specialist I see has a one-month or longer wait for new patients.

Good dentists take their time with patients. They do not rush the procedures and they make sure to perform each step carefully. That means that they will not be able to handle a large number of patients. Good dentists also get good referrals because they make people feel good. Their practices quickly fill up since there are so few good dentists. Good dentists usually do not have a full waiting room if they are the solo dentist in their practice, because they are not rushing from one patient to the next the way a typical medical doctor might. Good dentists care about the health of their patients, even if they do not say it. You can feel it. You will feel good after you leave the office of a good dentist.

Beyond the good dentists, there are great dentists, yet even they still make mistakes. They are human, and in the confines of the profession they may perform certain procedures very well, yet not excel at others. For example, one dentist might be brilliant with Endocal root canals, another might make great bridges, and another might be good at saving teeth or expertly using minimal drilling.

**Dental Referral Disclaimer:** Just because a dentist is on one of these lists does not mean that he or she performs completely non-toxic dentistry. It further does not mean that the dentists listed will all give you the best care, have only treatments that you agree with or that are beneficial for all people, or use the best biocompatible materials. Not every good dentist is on one of these lists, and not every dentist on these lists may be good for you. Using these lists is, however, a good way to significantly increase the chance of finding an excellent dentist. On some of these websites you will need to click around to find the referral pages.

**www.holisticdental.org**—The Holistic Dental Association

**www.toxicteeth.org**—Consumers for Dental Choice

**www.naturaldentistry.org**—The Institute for Nutritional Dentistry

**www.iabdm.org**—International Academy of Biological Dentistry

**www.hugginsappliedhealing.com**—Hal Huggins Trained Dentists

**www.iaomt.org**—International Academy of Oral Medicine and Toxicology

**www.dams.cc**—Dental Amalgam Mercury Solutions

**www.toothconservingdentistry.com**—Biomimetic Dentistry

# Finding a Dentist to Work with Diet

I have had people request that I refer them to dentists who work with diet who understand what I teach here in this book. There are some dentists who promote good nutrition, or healthy habits in alignment with this book, but they do not teach it or practice with it. If there are dentists who do, they generally keep to themselves. There are a few dentists trained by Dr. Huggins that can use blood tests to help you find your ancestral diet, which is based on the work of dentist Melvin Page. This is about as close as you will get to a dentist in alignment to the dietary principles presented in this book. In most cases a good solution is to get nutritional support from another natural health care provider and you can have your dentist monitor the health of your teeth.

## Minimally Invasive Dentistry

Minimally invasive dentists remove the least amount of tooth possible during a dental treatment. A conventional dentist drills and drills, removing significantly more tooth substance than is absolutely needed. Minimally invasive practices can also involve using lasers or other topical treatments that limit or prevent dental drilling. If drilling is needed, the best type of dentistry drills a small hole (lasers work well for this) and places a tiny composite filling in the hole. The integrity of the tooth is then maintained. Because of the precise cutting ability of lasers, laser dentistry can be minimally invasive. Lasers or air abrasion can also be done without pain killers and they avoid traumatizing the tooth from the vibration of the drill.

· · · · · · · · · · · · · · · · · · · · · · · · · · · · · · · · · · · · · · · · · · · · · · · · ·

### Non-Invasive Dentistry

If you have a small cavity, the non invasive dentist would advise you about the cavity curing power of cod liver oil. "Take two teaspoons per day, and come back next week."

Most cavities can be remineralized by diet alone.

· · · · · · · · · · · · · · · · · · · · · · · · · · · · · · · · · · · · · · · · · · · · · · · · ·

## Getting a Second Opinion

Five years ago, I had several painful spots on my teeth. I made an appointment with a dentist and x-rays were taken of my teeth. It felt terrible getting the x-rays because I felt their harmful effects. This dentist told me that I had four cavities to be filled. Strangely, the tooth that bothered me and the places where my teeth felt sensitive did not appear on the x-ray, and the dentist did not notice them in his examination. This dentist wanted to drill holes in teeth that were not painful. He did not notice, through examination or x-rays, where my tooth enamel was weak and where my teeth did hurt (I also did not tell him about the sensitive spots because I did not want to have more fillings placed). This occurred before I was educated about dentistry. I went to another dentist, at a community college, to get my teeth cleaned. This dentist had little profit motive because he was paid to teach dental hygienists and not to place fillings. He told me based on the same set of x-rays (which I brought from the first dentist) and through the same examination methods that I had one cavity. This dentist also said that I did not need to get it filled, but rather I should wait to see if it would improve. This is an amazing example of how money and the need for financial gain from performing dental surgery makes the dentist see cavities that are not really there. Money seems to make many dentists forget that not every cavity needs a treatment since it might remineralize and heal. Finally, a friend of mine who is a dentist told me, based on the same x-rays, that I had three cavities that needed to be filled, and showed them to me on the x-ray. I could clearly see one of the breaches in the tooth enamel in the x-ray. I was not really convinced that the two other ones even existed.

If you have any doubt in your dentist, get another opinion. Even if you totally trust your dentist, but you feel unsure of what to do next, get another opinion. If something your dentist says did not sound right to you, get another opinion. Trust that feeling inside of you that says, "Maybe I should get another opinion."

In case you are wondering, I no longer have any sensitive spots on my teeth. I have no evidence of tooth decay in my teeth, and I have not had a dental treatment on those teeth that had the putative cavities five years ago. My teeth feel strong and healthy. I have had digital x-rays examined by two different dentists, and today I do not have any cavities at all.

## Taking Charge at the Dentist's Office

There is a challenging interplay between being an informed patient, and trusting your dentist. On one hand you have good reason to know every bit of detail about what type of treatment your dentist is recommending. On the other hand, if you question every single move of your dentist to the point of paralyzing him in his treatment of your teeth, then he cannot perform his job in which he is skilled..

The dental office is a scary place. My best advice for taking charge at the dental office is to bring a friend. Now you have a witness. Call in advance to make sure your dentist accepts this. Since this is not a normal protocol except for parents and children, there may be some hesitancy on the dentist's part. Your friend can ask questions you did not think of, and watch your back in case you become disoriented from the dental procedures. Having a friend drive you to and from a dental procedure is also a good idea.

When you are in the dentist's office, share how you are feeling honestly. If you feel scared or unsure, let them know. Also try to state your boundaries upfront. Usually most of this can be done on the phone with the receptionist so you can avoid an uncomfortable situation in the first place. You can ask the receptionist such questions as, "I am looking for biocompatible treatments; does Dr. So-and-so perform blood serum compatibility testing, electrical or muscle testing?" When face to face with the dentist, tell them what you want and expect from them. Examples would be, "I want minimally invasive treatments; is that something you can do?" or "Please be upfront with what you think about my teeth so that I can choose the best treatment option based on your opinions."

Another approach is to set up a visit for a "consultation." Basically a consultation is when you pay the dentist for their time to diagnose your condition and to offer an opinion on what to do, but you are clear that you do not need or expect a treatment. Consultations are a good way to meet with a dentist and see how good they are based upon their diagnoses and suggestions for treatments. This can add up cost wise if you consult several dentists. It is also a good time to ask your dentist questions and to get educated while you are paying them for their time to talk. Consultations can be difficult to perform if you have a serious condition and just want the dentist's opinion. The dentist will want to follow their legal and perhaps moral obligations to treat you.

## Cavities and X-rays

One of my readers was overjoyed to have healed his gum problems. He then went to his conventional dentist for a check-up and was shocked when his dentist told him that one of his teeth needed a root canal. "How could this be?" he wondered, when the tooth felt fine. The dentist diagnosed the new cavity using older x-ray technology which can produce shadows or fuzzy images; these images showed a large black spot under one of his tooth fillings, which the dentist claimed was not in the previous x-ray taken 6 months prior. I advised the reader to seek care with a trusted holistic dentist. The holistic dentist used a more modern digital x-ray, which resulted in a clearer picture. The new x-ray showed no cavity at all. It turned out that the conventional dentist mistook a shadow from a tooth filling in the x-ray for a severe tooth cavity. The conventional dentist was obviously happy to show this reader his cavity, because he would make a nice profit for the week doing a root canal procedure. It is even possible his dentist knew that it was a shadow, but the potential for a large financial gain bypassed the dentist's reasoning process and had him see cavities that were not there. The conclusion I draw from this story and others like it is that there are likely tens of thousands, if not millions, of dental procedures being performed yearly that are totally unnecessary. Not only are they unnecessary from the perspective that they could be healed via nutrition, but fully unnecessary in that no condition exists that requires treatment.

In the case of a wrong diagnosis, once the dentist drills into your tooth he is not likely to say, "Whoops, I do not see any tooth decay; sorry to have drilled a huge hole in your tooth." Instead, he will keep on drilling, put that filling in, and pretend as though everything went as expected.

As readers of this book, you are now privileged with dental knowledge that I hope you will share with everyone: all of your relatives, friends, coworkers and second cousins. Then they too can learn how to avoid unnecessary dental procedures. Getting additional copies of *Cure Tooth Decay* and sharing is a good way to spread this knowledge. Sometimes dental procedures are a good idea, and that's when you want them; the rest of the time, you of course do not want them.

A good dentist should confirm his diagnoses with a second perspective. This means that an x-ray image should not be exclusively relied upon to make the decision to drill. Other testing methods include probing with an examiner, visual inspection, or using electrical or ultrasound tools to test the strength and health of the tooth.

## The Dental Code of Silence

The dental code of silence means that if a dentist sees bad dental work in a patient's mouth he will remain silent rather than enlighten his patient to his condition. The only time a dentist might comment on previous dental work is if it is extremely poorly done, and perhaps was performed in another country. The only thing we know from going to each dentist we visit is our experience of lying in the dental chair with our heads buzzing with the dental drill, and opening and closing our mouths to varying degrees. We have no idea if the dentist put in the most amazing and clean filling ever, or if he drilled away forever healthy tooth, and then placed the filling ineptly. I heard of a dentist who recently passed away. He would spend five hours working on one crown. He guaranteed his crowns would last 40 or more years. Quality dental work takes time.

The dentists' code of silence allows the profession to stay at low standards of performance since patients are not informed or educated about poor dental work versus good dental work. Bad dentists do not get caught, and they continue performing bad dental work. Mercury fillings are just another example of the dentists' code of silence. When dentists decline to take a stand against the tyranny of dental "ethics" boards that obfuscate the toxicity and harm caused by mercury fillings and toxic metals in the mouth, they allow the system to continue with impunity.

## *Root Canals*

George Meinig, DDS, was one of the founders of the American Association of Endodontists (root canal specialists). When he started in dentistry, everyone simply extracted decayed teeth. Dr. Meinig and other dentists had a great idea to save teeth rather than remove them if they were infected. Endodontists used to be on the fringe of dentistry and they worked hard to become mainstream specialists.

Now, each year in the U.S. alone there are more than 30,000,000 root canals performed. That is a 30 billion dollar industry. Dr. Meinig, once a root canal advocate after a lifetime of performing root canals as a dentist, changed his position after he read 1174 pages of detailed research by Dr. Weston Price and his 60-man research team. Meinig discovered that,

*A high percentage of chronic degenerative disease can originate from root filled teeth. The most frequent were heart and circulatory diseases. The next most common diseases were those of the joints, arthritis and rheumatism.*[241]

What Dr. Meinig urgently wanted to show people is that in many cases a root canal sets up the body for chronic and degenerative disease. If you have a significant degenerative condition, heart disease, severe headaches, arthritis and so forth, a root canal may be contributing to your condition or even to blame for it. The reason that root canals can be toxic is because each tooth contains about three miles of microscopic tubes. After a root canal procedure, the body's natural dentinal fluid flow to clean out the microscopic tubes is destroyed. A sick tooth can easily develop toxic substances within the microscopic tubules. It could be food particles or simply the death and putrefaction of the cells within the tiny tubes. This highly toxic substance can then drip down tiny fissures through the root of the tooth and enter your bloodstream. Dr. Price found that when bacteria could be filtered out of toxins extracted from root canals, that the toxin became more potent than when the bacteria were present. Bacteria from a root canalled tooth are not likely the cause of illness, but are simply feeding off and trying to clean up the rotting material. The conclusion of Dr. George Meinig's book *Root Canal Cover-Up* is that root canals are a really bad idea, and that they can be a serious source of disease.

Not all root canals become infected and not all root canals cause health problems. The most recent studies of root canal success rates over five- and ten-year periods reveal a dismal 30-40%. During the time of Dr. Price, the rate of root canals that definitely had no observable side effects was 25%.[242] Root canals present a catch-22 situation without any good choice. Root canals that are successful in the long run are going to be the ones that are not very infected before the treatment. These non-infected teeth are going to be the teeth that would have been the easiest to heal naturally and therefore did not really need root canals. The very damaged and rotten teeth are the ones that are the most difficult to heal and the most likely needing a root canal to save the tooth. These are cases where the root canal procedure will many times fail. Basically root canals work the best for the teeth that do not need them, and the worst for the teeth that do need them.

## Why People Have Tooth Infections

Your tooth became infected because it is weak and damaged. Material from your mouth environment entered deeply into the tooth, which is now inflamed. As a response to the foreign invader, the interior of the tooth acts to protect itself. This protection is known as an abscess. The body swells around the foreign material, and sends white blood cells to contain the material and dissolve it or to latch onto it and release it by collecting it in pus and then ejecting it out of your gums. The protective mechanism of your body is the swelling, which usually is accompanied by pain. The pain is an additional protection mechanism. Pain prevents you from chewing food in that location, so it minimizes the chances of more material entering into the weakened area. Pain also prevents you from chewing on the tooth so that it can be free from the biting pressure.

## What a Root Canal Procedure Accomplishes

A root canal is the complete removal of the guts of your tooth. A large hole is drilled into the top of your tooth, and the inner pulp of the tooth is removed. The inside of the tooth is then cleaned with chemicals. Once the inside is clean, a synthetic material is placed within the tooth, which is now partially dead, and a crown is placed on top of the tooth. If this crown has stainless steel or another metal in it, then you can have the problem of dissimilar metals in the mouth. It is really understandable why nobody is happy about root canals. They do not usually make you feel well.

With root canals, the dentist is manually accomplishing the cleansing of the interior of the tooth that your body has, due to imbalances, become incapable of doing for itself. Infections do not usually occur in healthy people; but if they do occur, the body quickly heals the infection. In unhealthy people, or people who are in moderate health but have a poor diet, infections cannot heal. Thus, a dentist is required to support their bodies in healing the infection. Infections also rarely occur in people who have a good bite, because correct bite places less stress upon teeth.

The problem with root canals is that the reason for the infection is not addressed. The cause of the infection could be a poor diet and an infection can loom up from below the root of the tooth, perhaps at first unseen. The tooth may be traumatized or damaged by excessive biting pressures. Cleaning out the guts of the tooth does not get to the root of the problem!

## Should You Remove A Root Canalled Tooth?

Nearly every root canalled tooth contains within it toxic material. In a minority of people, their body can wall off this source of infection, and they can be relatively unaffected by a root canal. If you suffer from serious or debilitating chronic health problems, consider seeing a professional who can help you determine if your root canals are causing your health problems. Infected root canals often go undetected by x-rays and can wreak havoc in the body. The danger of any root canal you already have is likely related to how unhealthy the tooth was in the first place. Root canals can be tested with a TOPAS test, electrical testing devices or muscle testing to help identify a root canal that is significantly harming your health.

The root canal procedure hides the pain of the infection, but usually it does not get down into the bone and tooth root tips where the infection may exist. The procedure also does not address the causative reason why the tooth is infected in the first place. Thus hidden infections can lurk at root canal sites.

If your health is not noticeably suffering, then many dentists believe you should keep your root canalled teeth.[243] Currently there is no real natural replacement for your tooth. And although we have the means to make healthy natural tooth replacements, I would not expect this technology to be available, successful, or affordable for at least 20 years. Once you remove your tooth there is no turning back.

Your bite and your ability to chew are supported by your tooth, even if it has a root canal. Numerous people have told me personally that they have regretted getting their root canalled teeth pulled because of how it affected their chewing or bite. An alternative to pulling a current tooth with root canal is to have your root canal resterilized with the newest technologies such as EndoCal 10. That being said, there is a time and place for certain root canalled teeth to be removed, and doing so has saved some people's lives.

## Safer Root Canals and Avoiding Root Canals at the Dental Office

EndoCal 10, formerly known as Biocalex is a form of calcium oxide. Holistically oriented dentists have reported good results from using this material. The root of the tooth needs to be carefully sealed up from toxins before this material is used.

As an alternative to a root canal, dentists can use the precision of a laser to vaporize infections in teeth without traumatizing the dental nerve.[244] This treatment can also save teeth from needing root canals or crowns. So rather than ripping the entire nerve of your tooth out, the dentist helps it heal and leaves it in place. Tooth infections can also be relieved sometimes by homeopathic injections to stimulate healing in a specific area of the jaw. These are much better ideas than root canals.

## Does Your Tooth Need a Root Canal?

A root canal is a heroic last resort treatment to spare removal of a tooth whose life has otherwise ended. A root canal is performed to clean up dangerous material and swelling that is not healing naturally. Without severe pain or inflammation, your tooth, while it may have a cavity, is still probably in relatively good health. So you do not want to remove the top of it and gut its insides unless there is no other option left.

A majority of root canals are unnecessary. I do not recommend or encourage the treatment. However in a case where there is absolutely no other choice, you will need to decide with your dentist and health practitioner if you want to try a carefully executed root canal or extract the tooth. If you are not in the situation of "there is no other choice," then you do not need a root canal. A root canal is not usually needed with cracked teeth that can be bonded together or in the case of inflamed areas near a tooth that could be a gum infection, not a tooth infection. If your tooth has never had a dental treatment, and it has not been severely traumatized then there is a very high likelihood that you do not need a root canal. If your tooth is inflamed, the inflammation can be treated with a good diet and herbs. Holistically oriented dentists also have tools to calm an infection, such as homeopathic injections and lasers to stimulate healing. If you have been told that you need a root canal but you do not feel any sort of pain, swelling or inflammation, then you more than likely do not need this dental treatment.

My concluding advice when considering whether to get a root canal is to ask yourself, "Does my body really need this treatment?" and, "Would a root canal contribute to my improved health?"

## How to Heal Tooth Inflammation or Tooth Infection (Tooth Abscess) and Avoid That Root Canal (these guidelines are not for children)

Many inflamed or infected teeth can heal naturally. But there are many cases where they cannot heal naturally and need the help of the dentist's hand to protect the tooth so that it can heal. In particular, teeth that are crowned, extensively traumatized, or with large mercury fillings can be very difficult to heal only with nutrition. This is because we are faced with a tooth that has suffered years and years of trauma. The trauma has come from biting forces, nighttime clenching or grinding, and a poor diet. After years and years of abuse, the tooth finally fails. It is a tall order to reverse a tooth that far gone with nutrition alone because it could take months to rebuild the structure of such a traumatized tooth.

The more suggestions you can follow on this list, the better your chances of healing a tooth infection in addition to following the previously presented dietary guidelines.

### Tooth Infection (Abscess) Healing Guidelines

1. Eat the tooth infection formula (chapter 6).

2. Take two teaspoons of cod liver oil, or Blue Ice™ Royal Blend per day.

3. Reduce biting forces by wearing a night guard.

4. Reduce biting stress by supplemental treatments including cranial osteopathy, chiropractic treatments on the jaw, acupressure, acupuncture, myofascial release, to name a few.

5. Avoid all grains.

6. Do not eat any fruit or sweets at all.

7. Use herbal topical treatments (see "Healing Tooth Pain" in this chapter).

8. Natto (special fermented soybeans) or the enzyme from natto, nattoki-
   nase increases blood circulation and can help reduce infections.

9. Prayer.

What is vital to understand here is that if you do have an infection, you are at a very delicate point with regard to your health. If the infection becomes more severe, which can happen rapidly if you are not careful, then your health is at risk. Please note that the success rate for curing a tooth infection will be lower than that for curing a cavity, as the infection is an indication of a more severe imbalance. Eating raw animal fats and proteins significantly increases the chance of healing the tooth infection.

If your health is otherwise compromised, such as if you have a chronic or debilitating disease, then please seek help from a minimally invasive dentist as the remedies here may not help you to a significant degree.

If you are taking the correct action, the tooth infection should not progress any further and the pain should not increase. You can expect a moderate improvement in 12–24 hours, and a more significant improvement with noticeable pain reduction in 24–48 hours. If you do not see this type of improvement, then you need immediate dental intervention.

## Understanding Tooth Infections

There are different types of infections so this description may not include the type of infection that you have. The phases of a tooth infection are:

1. Redness and swelling in the gums above the tooth.

2. Bumps or an additional swollen spot in gum above the tooth.

3. Small white ball of pus forming.

4. Large ball of pus in gum.

5. Swelling in face and neck.

6. Fever and severe swelling in face, neck and other parts of the body.

You can easily tell if you have an infection based upon the amount of pain you feel. Swelling and severe pain means a tooth infection. The infection can progress or regress through the different stages. When the infection is not visible, and cannot be seen on the x-ray, then the infection is gone from the perspective of requiring a dental treatment on a tooth. The infection still may linger hidden, but to effect a complete resolution of the infection would require herbs, diet, homeopathy and/or manual therapies.

### Tooth Infection Topical Treatments

The odds of curing tooth infections greatly increase when using supplemental herbal treatments.

1. **Plantain**—Place fresh, bruised plantain leaf directly on the infected and swollen area. Wild plantain is the best choice. To use plantain, chew it up and then place it on the inflamed area. Plantain has the action of pulling out dead and diseased material.

2. **Echinacea Tincture**—Place tincture of echinacea on the inflamed area. Echinacea has the ability to help heal infections. Also, it can be taken internally as described on the bottle.

3. **Potato for Abscess**—Place a slice of plain, white raw potato against the abscess, and leave in place for several hours.

# Focal Infections

The focal infection theory maintains that an infection in one place in the body can travel to and infect a distant place in the body. It is the spread of toxins from one part of the body through the bloodstream or by other means to another part. Focal infections have been proven to be connected with a large variety of health problems including blood problems, digestive problems, back pain, infertility, arthritis, abscess and infections throughout the body or on the skin, heart disease, allergies, kidney damage, brain tumors, cancer, trigeminal neuralgia and even death.[245]

Focal infections often times begin in the mouth. They are caused from inflamed gums, dead teeth particularly under root canals, and decaying jaw bone known as a NICO lesion. Hidden mouth infections can also reside in cavitations, which are holes in the bone often where a tooth—especially a wisdom tooth—has been extracted. This is a hidden area of pus, toxins or rotting bone. What happens is a part of the mouth is putrefying, or there are putrefied substances in places that the body cannot clean up at the tooth extraction site. I mention this condition because even if you eat well, you want to be sure that there is no rotting infectious material in your mouth causing disease in other parts of your body. I do not want people to live with untreated infections. You can treat many infections with nutrition. But some cases of infections will not heal properly just with nutrition particularly in the cases were the tooth is already damaged by dentistry with a large filling, crown or root canal. In these cases you will want good nutrition in combination with homeopathic injections or surgery to clean up and protect the area against infection.

### Tooth Extractions Because of Infections

Extracting teeth destabilizes the bite, weakens the jaw, and can lead to scar tissue formation.[246] Teeth are often extracted because of tooth infections, but the bone under the infected tooth is many times not cleaned up after the extraction. This can then become a source of a focal infection and lead to chronic pain such as hip and back pain along with migraine headaches.[247] In my opinion, because of the importance of having a functional bite, teeth should only be extracted as an absolute last resort when medically necessary and it should not be a standard treatment for any sort of tooth infection.

# Dental Implants

The post of a dental implant allows a space for toxins to enter into the gum because the periodontal ligament and gum tissue do not attach to the implant sufficiently to seal off that space. There is hardly any evidence available regarding the long-term effects of titanium implants. Placing metal directly into the jaw bone poses a high risk of triggering a negative immune system reaction in the patient.[248] The body reacts poorly to any implanted metal. Studies at the Karlinska Institute in Sweden, show that most humans become rapidly allergic to virtually any metal placed inside the human body including mercury, titanium and gold. One not commonly considered problem with titanium implants is the battery effect of combining titanium with other metals from dental restorations in your mouth.

Zirconium is a non metal material that is used for implants in other modern parts of the world. It has been recently approved for use in the United States. If you decide you want an implant, for the same cost as having a titanium implant here, you can fly to another country such as New Zealand and get a zirconium implant there.

As with any dental procedure, you must weigh the benefits and the costs to determine if this is right for you. Clearly we want to place our efforts into keeping our existing teeth because none of the alternatives are fully satisfactory, and they are costly.

# Dental Abuse

With a few exceptions, modern dentistry is an inhumane system. Many dentists coerce patients into treatments that they do not need. Part of this system of coercion is to first condemn patients as failures in life because they did not prevent their tooth decay due to poor oral hygiene. These accusations can weaken patients' sense of self and get them to succumb to unneeded dental procedures. You know a dentist has abused you if you feel sick or awful in their presence, or if they try to coerce you into treatments that you feel unsure about. A majority of dentists are in business to make money. And the business aspect has corrupted most dentists so surely and thoroughly, it causes them to behave in irresponsible ways.

Dental abuse is also physical abuse because dental treatments when not absolutely needed damage and harm your physical body. Dental treatments that use toxic metals cause disease, pain, and suffering. This is also a form of physical abuse, and it is unethical.

## Suggestions for Healing Dental Abuse

1. **Acknowledge the past trauma** that has been inflicted on your teeth when you did not know any better. Feel it as fully as you can. Feel how upset, disoriented, taken advantage of, unfairly treated or numbed you feel. Let those feelings have a space or a voice. Feel the profound suffering that dentistry is causing people. Look it squarely in the eye.

2. **Forgive.** Once the problem is acknowledged then ask for healing and forgiveness. Is there any way you can find that tiny spark in yourself that is capable of forgiving yourself for being a victim, and forgiving the dentist for his extreme ignorance and arrogance? By the way, forgiveness does not mean you do not hold the dentist or dentistry in general responsible for their negligent behavior.

3. **Get educated.** Once you are able to let go of some of the past attachments towards dentistry, then it is time to learn about good dentistry that can repair toxic dentistry. Seek out dentists who practice less toxic and minimally invasive dentistry.

4. **Educate your friends and family.** Healing the abuse of dentistry means your community needs to be educated about the severe problems with conventional dentistry. Part of your own healing from dental abuse will come by educating your friends and family about the dangers and hazards prevalent in dentistry.

On the practical side, if you do not feel good at your dentist's, then speak up. If you still feel confused and unsure, leave the dental office immediately. Get a second opinion.

# *Do I Have a Cavity?*
# *Understanding Tooth Decay*

A cavity is an impairment in the tooth structure that creates sensitivity to the environmental forces in the mouth such as saliva, foods, and chewing. A cavity is any structural weakness in a tooth that causes the tooth to function improperly. Feeling pain, discomfort, finding white spots and sometimes black spots on your tooth, having hot or cold sensitivity, and not wanting to chew on a tooth are the results of tooth decay. For a majority of people the simplest way to know if you have a cavity is to go to a good dentist for a check-up. For the minority of people, you can do it at home. Most people are better off working with a dentist because dentists have the experience needed to clearly diagnose cavities. This is where a dentist can be your ally.

The guidelines below will give you a general idea of the type of tooth problems you are facing. These suggestions are not guaranteed to accurately diagnose your problems, but they can aid you in understanding your experience. **If you need a more accurate diagnosis then please seek professional dental help.**

> *Tooth Pain: Temporary sensitivity to hot or cold foods, without recent dental work.*
> **Meaning:** Tooth decay is active. The tooth enamel is weak and sensations travel more rapidly to the nerve. This may also be the beginning signs of gum disease.

> *Tooth Pain: Lasting sensitivity and more constant awareness of hot or cold foods, without recent dental work.*
> **Meaning:** The tooth pulp could be infected, the tooth may be cracked or chipped, or this is the beginning of gum disease.

> *Tooth Pain: Temporary sensitivity to hot or cold foods after a recent dental treatment.*
> **Meaning:** Dental work can cause tooth pulp inflammation, which would be an intense but very brief pain. The tooth pulp should heal within 2-4 weeks of a dental treatment.

> *Tooth Pain: Lasting or prolonged sensitivity and constant awareness of hot or cold foods after a recent dental treatment.*
> **Meaning:** The cavity may have been too close to the tooth pulp so the dental treatment did not protect the pulp sufficiently. This is a common and unfortunate problem from imprecise dental work or too much drilling.

**Tooth Pain:** *Sharp pain from biting down on food.*
**Possible Meanings**: Loose filling, tooth decay, cracked or fractured tooth, infected tooth.

**Tooth Pain:** *Constant and severe pain with pressure, swelling of the gum, and sensitivity to touch.*
**Meaning:** Tooth or gum abscess (tooth infection).

**Pain:** *The tooth hurts when you tap it with your finger from the side.*
**Meaning:** The periodontal ligament is degenerating or inflamed.

**Tooth Pain**: *Dull ache, headaches, tooth experiences lingering hot-cold sensitivity that lasts much longer than a few seconds.*
**Meaning**: The tooth nerve is damaged or dying. There may be a hidden infection.

**Tooth decay** *that occurs on the top of teeth, or dental tartar.*
**Meaning:** Too much free calcium in your blood, the calcium is not being used efficiently. The form of calcium may be unabsorbable.

**Tooth decay** *that is near or below the gum line, or red, tender or inflamed gums.*
**Meaning**: Too much free phosphorous in your blood; your body is not using phosphorous efficiently. This could also be from excess biting forces causing stress on the roots of the tooth.

# Monitoring Tooth Decay and Tooth Remineralization

I encourage readers to monitor tooth decay with their dentist. While it is not necessary to work with a dentist if you would rather not, I do find that bringing the awareness and skills of a trusted dentist into the picture can greatly help you. When you monitor the progress of tooth decay carefully you can determine whether or not the dietary changes you have implemented are helping your teeth. If the dietary changes are not helping, you need to make more changes or consider dental surgery. Examining your teeth frequently helps you stay aware of the reality of your dental health. The programs in this book are not about just eating healthy food while remaining oblivious to the effectiveness of the protocol. This is about being mindful of your dental health and paying attention to any changes that might occur. Clear digital x-rays can show convincing documentation when tooth dentin is remineralizing.

Dentists check for tooth decay by examining x-rays and by using a tool called an explorer. With the explorer, the dentist probes for soft or sticky spots in the teeth. He also will check around the neck of the tooth for hidden root cavities.

There are various methods for you to monitor your tooth remineralization, and people have employed different strategies. One way to monitor your tooth decay is to eat a small amount of certain foods, or drink hot or cold water, that typically cause tooth pain. Another is to press your teeth in various spots with your fingernail. If you want to be more precise, you can purchase a dental explorer at the local drug store and use it carefully in the same way. If you feel a soft spot or experience tooth pain while using the dental explorer, then you have tooth decay. Decayed spots are usually slightly sticky or feel like rotten wood. Some dentists offer a saliva test to determine if tooth decay is active. Using these tests, you can check and monitor the progress of your dietary changes, watching to see whether or not your tooth is getting harder.

I also encourage you to do a visual inspection of your teeth. You can accomplish this by using an efficient light and the bathroom mirror. A small dental mirror can also be useful for inspecting your teeth from different angles. A visual inspection can help you determine if your teeth are healthy. Take a digital photograph of your teeth if possible, and label them for comparison.

You are to be responsible for monitoring your dental health. I support active participation in your dental recovery program. I do not encourage excessive x-rays because of the dangers of radiation exposure. Digital x-rays emit less radiation than conventional ones, but they still emit some. By checking your progress, you will be able to determine whether or not the diet you are following is working and you will be able to catch a problem before it becomes worse.

## *Understanding Tooth Remineralization*

Your body is always trying to heal and repair your teeth to find and maintain balance. I described this previously as *vis medicatrix naturae*. Your goal is to align yourself and your actions with this natural function. Any tooth has the potential to remineralize. If healing teeth seems confusing, just think of bones healing. Healing teeth is similar to healing bones. When your diet reaches a certain threshold of minerals and fat-soluble vitamins, your soft teeth will turn hard and even glassy. Cracks can seal together, and your tooth ligaments will strengthen. Inside the tooth your body will build new secondary dentin to protect the inner tooth pulp. As with a bone, if there is a hole in your tooth, the hole will not usually fill in. The areas all around the hole will get strong and extremely hard. The lost tooth structure is not usually replaceable. Holes in your teeth usually cannot be completely filled in and restored to their original condition, even with special nutrition. However, the holes can be sealed, and the enamel will become hard and protect your tooth pulp from infection.

# *How to Treat Your Decayed Tooth*

I frequently am asked about what to do in specific instances of decayed teeth. My answer is very simple. Do the best you can with nutrition. And then evaluate with your dentist if your tooth needs further cosmetic or surgical treatments. It never hurts to improve your diet in any case.

What to do about your tooth decay depends on how severe it is. The severity is determined by how much pain you experience, if there is a large visible cavity in the tooth, and if the tooth has been drilled or traumatized in the past. Understanding the past condition of the tooth will guide you to what type of treatments your tooth needs under a diet that promotes tooth remineralization such as described in this book. The advice here is meaningless for those who neglect to carefully ensure that they have enough fat-soluble vitamins in their diet while avoiding many of the tooth-decay-promoting foods.

Dental problems in teeth that have been drilled by dentists usually need to be repaired in some way by a good dentist. The model of drilling large holes guided by the "extension for prevention" premise traumatizes teeth. The tooth with a moderate to large mercury filling has lost its structural strength from the large hole drilled in it. Some older composite fillings may also exhibit this loss of structural integrity if they are weakly bonded to the tooth. An analogy for these sorts of teeth is a house without a roof. Without a sound roof, any kind of foul weather will be able to enter the house. The house will be hard to clean, and likely will be damaged from the weather. Likewise, your tooth that has been drilled is like a house without a roof. Your body has to work tremendously hard to clean, repair, and maintain the damaged tooth because it has little protection from the environment of your mouth. If your house did not have a roof, would it make sense to continue to try to clean it up after every rain or snow? No. It would make sense to fix the roof to prevent the problem in the first place. Likewise, bad dentistry needs to be fixed with good dentistry. Teeth that have mercury fillings, toxic crowns, or conventional root canals are like houses without roofs.

With teeth that have already been subject to the dentist's drill, no matter what the condition of the tooth, be it painful, temperature sensitive, cracked, or infected your treatment path will require the work of the tooth handyman, the dentist. Great dentists can bond teeth, save inflamed nerves, and restore the structural integrity of your tooth with carefully bonded ceramics or composites. Once the tooth is safe and not being traumatized it can heal faster. The tricky part is that if you go to a dentist with a large amount of tooth decay, then he usually will want to remove all of the decayed part of the tooth, even part of the tooth that can remineralize. How long you wait to remineralize the tooth, how much the dentist needs to drill, if at all, and if you should have a temporary or permanent filling placed while the tooth heals is all entirely up to you to decide along with, one hopes, the supportive advice from your dentist.

Teeth that have never been drilled usually respond very well to dietary intervention. You should notice significant improvement in tooth pain or sensitivity within a few days. Once the tooth has hardened then you can decide with your dentist if the tooth needs extra structural support from a filling. In this case you could do a no-drill filling if there was a large hole that needed to be sealed up. I do not recommend leaving large holes untreated, although some people make this choice for personal reasons. Tiny cavities, the kind most people have, do not really need any type of drilling or filling once they remineralize. All that is there will usually be a tiny but very hard discolored or black spot on the tooth. Sometimes even the discoloration of a cavity disappears completely on an excellent diet.

With your excellent diet your tooth will now be constantly trying to heal itself. If your dental condition has been going on for years and years, it could take many weeks or even many months to fully remineralize the damaged tooth. If your tooth is constantly getting aggravated such as from night time tooth clenching, tooth grinding, a poor bite, or dental work that is falling apart then the healing process is going to be very slow if it progresses at all. Meanwhile if your tooth is in a lot of pain, it may be difficult or impossible to wait for weeks and months for your body to heal the tooth nutritionally to the point where it stops hurting. The only way to know is to implement as much as you can of the tooth infection program explained earlier in this chapter. If your painful, inflamed tooth does not radically improve in 24–48 hours, then this tooth likely needs a dental treatment.

## Specific Examples of How to Treat Tooth Decay

Assuming you have changed your diet for the better, your teeth will be getting hard and strong. There may still be holes and these will become covered over with hard new enamel, but will not usually fill in. The general treatment theory on teeth is that less is more. You want to do the least traumatizing and least invasive treatment as is reasonable for your tooth. The best holistically oriented dentists will be able to support this process. What the least invasive treatment looks like exactly in your case you will need to decide for yourself. When people ask me what they should do with their tooth condition, I always simply ask them what they want to do. Beyond the structure of health I provide in this book, I cannot tell you or advise you what to do with your teeth. I cannot replace your own wisdom and inner knowing of what is right for you. Here I will try to give you some guidelines to help you make a good decision.

Soft leathery decay probably cannot be remineralized, but all of the other types of tooth decay can be remineralized. Your dentist will advise a specific filling or treatment for your tooth based upon his observation of how damaged the tooth is. If the decay is very hard, then the dentist should not need to drill much or at all. All cavity treatments and outcomes will be enhanced when you make steps to correct your bite and to relieve pressure on the central cranial nerve in your jaw, the trigeminal nerve. This will be discussed in the next chapter. Healing teeth nutritionally is enhanced by topical treatments including herbs, homeopathy, sea salt rinses, gum cleaning and oil pulling (see the gum disease chapter).

**Side Cavities and Regular Cavities**. These respond well to nutritional adjustments. After the small cavity has healed, you will need to decide if you want or need any additional drill-free dental treatments to restore the structure or look of the particular tooth.

**Large cavity**. Make dietary changes and then get the cavity filled with a no-drill filling, or a filling that requires only a small amount of drilling. This can only be done when the cavity is remineralized. Alternatively, the cavity can be scraped carefully without using a drill and then a temporary or permanent filling can be placed while you improve your diet. Teeth can remineralize under the fillings. Parts of the teeth that are drilled are a far larger obstacle to tooth remineralization than a filling sitting in a tooth.

**Cavities under fillings.** Sometimes these respond well to nutrition, and other times they do not. It depends on how stressed the tooth is, and how severe the decay. First you need to determine if your current filling is allowing food and saliva to enter deeply into the tooth. If so, you want to get the filling cleaned, and then sealed with either a temporary or a permanent filling. If the filling on the tooth is already sound, then the first thing to consider is if this is a misdiagnosis. If it is not a misdiagnosis, many of these teeth will respond well to nutritional treatments. Make sure to avoid biting on the tooth as best as you can for 1–14 days depending on your desires, and perhaps even wear a night guard to relieve the nighttime stress on the tooth. Expect significant improvement in these deep cavities in 1–2 weeks. If the filling is damaged, once the interior of the tooth heals, then consider getting a new non-toxic filling to strengthen the structure of your tooth.

**Cracked or chipped teeth**. Cracking teeth is almost always a sign of a significant dietary sin or health imbalance. Teeth are not supposed to crack, even in the elderly. Whole grains and high intensity sweeteners top the list of dietary mistakes that cause cracking or chipping. Cracked teeth can usually be bonded by a good dentist. You will need to reduce the biting stress on the tooth and give it ample time to heal. To reduce biting stress a night guard, chewing on the opposite side, and alternative body work treatments on your jaw or head will help. Just as a reminder, a cracked or chipped tooth does not usually need a root canal.

**Teeth with temporary fillings**. You will want to find a permanent safe filling solution and not keep temporary fillings in your mouth very long.

**Leaving big cavities without fillings.** A few daring people want to have no filling materials in their mouths even if their teeth have large holes. I do not recommend this option if you are doing it to save money.

**A mouth full of cavities, or you do not know what to do about your cavities.** What I always say to people who feel unsure is to make your best effort to improve your diet. No matter what dental treatment course you pursue, you will always be benefited by improving your diet. It does not hurt to try.

**Sensitivity on sides of teeth with gum line ridges.** This is called abfraction and is due to biting forces. An improved diet will strengthen the tooth against the loss or damage to the tooth caused by biting forces. The complete healing of this condition may require additional treatments to adjust how you bite.

# Still not Sure? Talk to Your Tooth

While this suggestion may sound ridiculous, I assure you that I have not gone off the deep end! I want you to know that I am sharing this suggestion with you because many people truly have difficulty in deciding how to take care of a painful tooth, and this process really can bring clarity.

Even after considering all of this information, you still might feel clueless about what to do for your painful tooth. You may wonder if there is any hope. Many times in these situations you have a variety of choices. And it requires relaxing the judgmental mind to know which choice is best for you.

Consider beginning an inner dialog with your tooth. This is very similar to talking with a child. Here are some examples. "How are you, tooth?" "What will make you feel better?" "Do you want to visit a dentist?" "Do you want a root canal?" "Do you want to try herbs?" "Do you want a special food?" "Do you want to be pulled?" You will be amazed at how your body can actually communicate what it needs to you. People will receive some kind of response to these questions, as a feeling, an inner knowing or voice, or as a desire to do something. If you get no response, do not worry. A response will appear in some way when your mind is relaxed. Keep asking clearly. A treatment option can also elicit a feeling of stress or tension (implying it is a bad choice), and a feeling of lightness and ease in response to another treatment (implying this is a good choice). If this exercise is too abstract, place an object near you to represent your hurting tooth. Then talk to the object as if it is your tooth. This can be therapeutic and help you to discern what is best to do. For example, you could express some anger, sadness, disappointment or frustration at your tooth, or at yourself, for hurting. If you can let yourself have some fun here, then you might get an insight on how to proceed.

. . . . . . . . . . . . . . . . . . . . . . . . . . . . . . . . . . . . . . . . . . . . . . . . . .

**Dental Mystery—Missing Adult Teeth**

About 3% of the population exhibits a condition in which some of the primary or permanent teeth are missing. This condition is called hypodontia, and is associated with genetic or environmental factors. Problems with primary and adult teeth not erupting have been shown in cases of rickets, syphilis, and in laboratory animal experiments with a very high sugar diet. Congenital syphilis is linked to missing teeth. Its symptoms on the skeletal system are very similar to that of scurvy and rickets.[249] Scurvy in children was treated with raw minced beef, fresh cow's milk, and orange juice. Perhaps missing teeth is related to a lack of vitamin C or a lack of fat-soluble vitamin D in the diet during important times of growth including in the womb. The exact cause of missing teeth still remains a mystery.

. . . . . . . . . . . . . . . . . . . . . . . . . . . . . . . . . . . . . . . . . . . . . . . . . .

# The Vicious Cycle and Tooth Decay

One school of thought proposes that emotions are the primary cause of physical disease. Another school of thought declares the opposite, citing that disease has little to do with emotions. Let us try to clear up this mess so you can take care of your teeth in the healthiest way possible.

Emotions and stress can absolutely affect your health. The way your emotions affect your health is primarily through poor food choices when you feel bad, or unhappy, and good food choices when you feel well. Emotions such as sadness, anger, and grief can also interfere with your body's ability to digest food.

Emotions do affect your internal body chemistry which can alter your calcium and phosphorous balance. Strong emotions can engage the fight or flight response within your glands (adrenal, pituitary, thyroid and so on). The fight or flight response will cause poisonous substances to be secreted into your blood stream readying you for attack or to run for your life. While many situations in our modern lives feel like fight or flight events, the reality for most people is that **we do not live in truly life or death situations in our modern world.** Many people behave as if they do, but this is an artificially created reality that is in part exaggerated by the mass media. If you behave as if every news event, traffic jam, or bad look from a stranger is the end of your life, then your body is going to use up tremendous amounts of resources for nothing.

I have noticed that some people who experience severe tooth decay are severely stressed. They are in a hurry, always rushing, putting their needs off until the last minute. When someone comes to me and they cannot slow down, take a breath, and just take a look at themselves for a moment, then I know they most likely will fail in remineralizing tooth decay. This is what is known as the vicious cycle. Difficult events challenge us in life, and rather than getting easier, life sends us more difficult events. The cycle also works constructively for certain people in certain parts of their lives, such as the person who always gets one good job or economic fortune after the next.

Your job is to transform the negative cycle of dental health into a positive cycle. The way this happens is by inviting in the positive feelings and experiences, while at the same time searching for and acknowledging the negative experiences. Stress is primarily caused by unacknowledged feelings. In modern society, we face life situations that our bodies are physically and emotionally unequipped for, such as eating a sandwich while driving and talking on a cell phone at the same time. As a result, we experience this specific kind of uncomfortable tension we call stress. To help deal with stress, one must slow down, breathe, and acknowledge the feelings present in this moment. The simple question of, "What is here now?" helps bring one's focus into the moment. One could also ask, "How am I feeling now?" These are some tools that help enhance awareness. Yoga, meditation, tai chi, chi gong, and many other forms of meditation, movement, or therapy, will help you reduce stress, clear your mind, and make you a healthier person.

Just relax and trust the healing process for your teeth. This means trusting you will be fine, whether you get a dental treatment on the tooth or not. Feel, or imagine a positive feeling of support that you can overcome tooth decay. If you have a negative doubting voice, just notice it and smile at it.

Through dedicated yoga practice, I began noticing how my body was being negatively affected by the food I ate. (I was eating foods on the "avoid" list before I knew any better, particularly "health food bars" and tofu.) This encouraged me to improve my diet. I became keenly aware of the physical consequences of poor food choices. Even today, I closely monitor my diet and stay disciplined so I do not succumb to negative food habits from the past. I also encourage you to review the beginning of chapter about healing children's cavities for more pointers on dealing with feelings.

## The Hidden Need to Be Sick

You may find this section difficult to believe. I bring it up here because I want to challenge you to be at your best to heal your teeth. As much as people want healthy teeth, very few people actually have a 100% whole-hearted desire or intention to be healthy. An experienced health practitioner opened my book to this page and exclaimed how so many of her patients actually wanted to be sick.

Most of us have a mixed bag of emotions in relation to our intention to be healthy. Just like the moon, we have our own light side and our own dark side. Yet when we just focus on our light side, and ignore the dark side, we are missing out on what makes life beautiful and balanced. The light part of us wants to be healthy and the dark side wants to be unhealthy. The classic result of this inner conflict is wishing our tooth decay to be fixed, without wanting to do any of the work to fix it. This is a key belief that has given rise and power to modern dentistry. Dentistry helps us not face our dark side that wants to be sick. Conventional dentistry allows us to be sick by telling us that we have nothing to do with tooth decay, that it is all the action of the bacteria and what the bacteria eat.

The result of the missing dark side of yourself that only pops up here and there when nobody is looking, is that we might subconsciously equate being healthy with suffering. The suffering associated with the effort needed to become healthy can manifest in many forms: complaining about exercise, believing in disempowering information, or not wanting to pay extra for healthy foods or a better dentist. These behaviors are a result of the interplay between your light side that wants to get healthy, and your dark side that does not care or that does not want health.

Putting more commitment and energy behind your goal of health requires positive feelings, beliefs and good will. If you are not fully committed to this positive result, then there must be some hidden negativity. This hidden dark side feels as though it has to suffer. It does not want the best. The dark side can make it hard for you to take care of yourself. To help transform the dark side you cannot simply ignore it and push it away. That would merely create more darkness. Just as there is nothing wrong with the dark side of the moon, your own dark side is not bad; it is simply a part of life that needs to be accepted. The way to cause a transformation is to bring light (awareness) to the darkness (unconsciousness). To help heal this hidden internal dilemma, I suggest three things:

1. Acknowledge and look for the unconscious wish to not live, or to not be healthy.

2. Meditate upon, or pray for help, or discuss with friends your dark side. Look for ways to bring the dark side into the light.

3. Commit to excellence. Without force, see if you are willing to make the simple commitment that "I want the best for myself," or "I deserve the best in life."

Making a new commitment to yourself or to life is the first step towards breaking the vicious cycle of tooth decay. Then you can start to see the hidden gold of your suffering, and that there are important lessons, meaning and purpose in your life, if you are willing to embrace them.

## *Busting the Myth that Food-Stuck-On-Teeth Causes Cavities*

Dentists, it is time to give up this arcane concept that carbohydrates fermenting on teeth are eaten by acid-producing bacteria that cause tooth decay. This theory is akin to saying that rain causes your roof to leak. When the roof of your home is sealed and well cared for it will not leak whether it rains or not. Likewise when your tooth enamel is strong and healthy your teeth will not be affected by the changing conditions in your mouth. W.D. Miller, the originator of the bacterial theory of tooth decay, said it himself in 1883, "What we might call the perfect tooth *would resist indefinitely* the same acid to which a tooth of opposite character would succumb in a few weeks." Because bacteria are everywhere, trying to eliminate bacteria from your mouth to prevent tooth decay would be like trying to eliminate rain from the sky to prevent a leaky roof.

Many of the cultures Dr. Weston Price studied relied upon a significant portion of their diet from carbohydrates including milk and carbohydrate-rich grain products, yet suffered practically no tooth decay. The healthy Gaelic people of the Outer Hebrides, who ate approximately 1000 calories of properly prepared oats per day, had almost no tooth decay (0.7–1.3% of all teeth affected). The isolated Swiss of the Loetschental Valley, who ate approximately 800 calories per day of properly prepared rye bread, had little evidence of tooth decay (0.3%–5.2% of all teeth affected). The 5.2% figure comes from the Visperterminen region where both potatoes and wine were used; the other isolated Swiss, with higher immunity to cavities, did not use wine and may not have used potatoes. The isolated Swiss, with near total immunity to tooth decay, did not even use toothbrushes, and had typical deposits of food on their teeth all the time without any tooth decay.

Indigenous people throughout the world did not typically brush or floss. Dr. Price comments on the impossibility of keeping teeth clean by brushing and flossing:

> *Among the difficulties in applying this interpretation is the physical impossibility of keeping teeth bacteriologically clean in the environment of the mouth. Another difficulty is the fact that **many primitive races have their teeth smeared with starchy foods almost constantly** and make no effort whatsoever to clean their teeth. **In spite of this they have no tooth decay.**[250] (Emphasis added.)*

The theory that bacteria in our mouth produce acids, which then cause tooth decay, is a false conclusion. Saliva has a basic pH and will neutralize acids in the mouth rather rapidly. The digestive enzymes in our saliva rapidly dissolve carbohydrates in our mouths. For example, bread can turn into liquid after being chewed several times. By the way, this section was not written to encourage people to abandon cleaning their teeth and mouths. The practice of dental and oral hygiene has many social benefits.

# *Tooth Care*

## Healing Tooth Pain

When the nutritional program is successful, tooth pain will decrease and teeth will feel firmer in your mouth. In some cases your teeth will need extra help as fast as possible. The following treatments are not full remedies, but rather intermediate treatments that help stop tooth pain. Here are seven of the most successful treatments for halting tooth pain. Each treatment can stand alone, or you can try several of them together.

1. Place clove oil or powdered cloves on the painful tooth.

2. Swish organic sesame seed or coconut oil in your mouth for 5-10 minutes and then spit it out. This is called oil pulling and is also a good method for cleansing the body and improving oral health.

3. Place goldenseal powder on or near the painful tooth.

4. Place oil of oregano on the tooth.

5. Dissolve a moderate amount of natural salt in a small amount of water and swish it in your mouth for at least one minute. Repeat several times throughout the day.

6. Echinacea, also known as the "toothache plant," can be applied topically on the tooth and/or taken internally using the tincture or powdered form.

7. Supplementing with vitamin $B_5$, pantothenic acid. Food sources rich in $B_5$ include: liver, sunflower seeds, shiitake mushrooms and eggs.

## Dental Sealants

Many dental sealants contain hormone-altering chemicals, including bisphenol A.[251] There are two purported less-toxic approaches; one is a resin sealant made by Ultradent, and the other is a glass ionomer sealant. The problem with resin sealants is that they do not allow minerals or fluids to pass through the surface of the tooth, thus inhibiting the dentin fluid flow. Glass ionomer sealants do allow the fluid to flow through the sealant. Due to the curing time needed to set the sealant, they are difficult to place properly and ideally should be done one tooth per visit. If a tooth already has a cavity, then putting a sealant on top of the tooth cavity will not help. This means that each tooth has to be carefully tested with a device such as a Diagnodent™ to search for small hidden pockets of tooth decay. Sealants do not block out decay completely but merely slow the process down, assuming they are placed properly. My conclusion is that sealants will benefit people in special situations as long as they avoid ones with hormone altering chemicals. In general, unless you feel really inspired to get a sealant, it seems unnecessary.

### Teeth Cleaning at the Dentist

One of the most common questions people ask me is if they need to get their teeth cleaned at the dentist. As to many of the questions people ask me, my response is that it is your choice. There is nothing you ever **have to** do. The question to start asking yourself is, "Is this in the best interests of my health?" The purpose of a teeth cleaning done by the dentist or hygienist is to remove the plaque and deposits on and around the tooth. My personal experience is that having my teeth scaled with the metal probe is extremely uncomfortable.

A better question is whether tooth cleaning improves dental health, or if positive aspects of tooth cleaning outweigh the negative. In my personal experience, after having my teeth cleaned with an ultrasonic cleaner, my body felt lighter. Since I am now using an oral irrigator and the blotting technique, along with continued improvements in my digestive health I hope to not need any cleanings in the future. I personally avoid the metal probe teeth scraping and cleaning. Any type of cleaning, scaling or ultrasonic, has the potential to hyperstimulate the nerves in your teeth and jaw.[252]

There is clear evidence that tooth brushing may cause slight wear to teeth in some cases even without toothpaste. The abrasiveness of toothpaste in combination with tooth brushing can definitely cause damage to the tooth enamel.[253] So the concept that enamel is as hard as diamonds and nothing can damage it is false. If small amounts of grit in toothpaste can damage tooth enamel, then it would seem absolutely clear that tooth cleaning using force and sharp metal probes will definitely in some cases scratch tooth enamel. At this time I am unable to locate specific evidence in the dental literature to prove that tooth cleaning with a metal probe is either safe or dangerous.

## Teeth Whitening At the Dentist's and At Home

Healthy indigenous people had naturally white teeth, even without brushing. One reader after reading my book went off of sugar for one year. By the end of that year time period, the reader's teeth went from yellowish to bright white. Not everyone gets very white teeth from following the advice in this book. Teeth are discolored for two key reasons. One reason is foods eaten can stain the teeth, for example, herbs, black tea or coffee. Another type of tooth discoloring is yellow teeth. I believe this is a form of tooth jaundice. This basically means that your body is a bit toxic, and your liver is not functioning optimally. As your liver gets healthier with a healthier diet, exercise, and therapeutic treatments like herbs, your teeth may gradually get whiter.

There are a variety of teeth whitening treatments available at your dentist. Some of them are relatively safe, while others remove healthy tooth structure. Based on the principle of choosing the least invasive treatment to your teeth as possible, you should avoid any tooth whitening material that contains any type of acidic or etching compound, and avoid all types of porcelain laminates. Avoid any whitening procedure that involves any drilling or removal of healthy enamel. Request your dentist, before submitting to any tooth whitening procedures, use no acid or etching materials.

## Natural Tooth Whitening

Dab a small amount of organic peppermint essential oil on your finger (much less than a drop), rub your finger on your toothbrush, and then brush normally. Some people might find that organic tea tree oil provides wonderful benefits. Another suggestion is charcoal. Keep in mind some of these methods are slightly abrasive to teeth.

**Dental Tip for Whiter Teeth**
To naturally remove stains and whiten teeth polish your teeth using a wet cotton swab dipped in baking soda. With a bit of pressure, rub the tooth enamel only, avoiding the gums. This tip was provided from Rupam who makes a great tooth soap. Learn more at: www.RupamHerbals.com

# Brushing, Flossing and Toothpaste

When the tooth surface is weak, then keeping the oral environment clean definitely is a good idea. My personal experience has been that a clean oral environment is helpful in reducing the impact of tooth decay. Cleaning your teeth helps prevent cavities when the dentinal fluid is flowing in the wrong direction. In this situation of demineralization, substances from within your mouth can enter into the tooth. Cleaning teeth will change the environment of your mouth and it can help slow down the problem, but it does not stop the original cause of tooth decay. If cleaning teeth did stop cavities, then why does 90% of our population get cavities?

## Toxic Toothpaste

Many brands of toothpaste contain the following warning. "WARNING: Keep out of the reach of children under 6 years of age. If you accidentally swallow more than used for brushing, seek professional assistance or contact a Poison Control Center immediately." If something is that dangerous where more than a tiny amount is considered poison, then I do not want to be putting it in my body every day.

Toothpaste is regulated as a cosmetic product, and not as a food. I suppose the rationale behind this is that toothpaste is not swallowed and that it does not get absorbed into your body. As a result the standards of safety for toothpaste are much lower than our already very low safety standards for food additives. Since toothpaste is not a food, almost anything goes as far as ingredients are concerned. Toothpastes usually contain ingredients like hydrated silica, sorbitol, sodium saccharin, titanium dioxide, glycerin, sodium lauryl/laureth sulfate, and sodium fluoride.

**Hydrated silica** is made from quartz and sand and it is an abrasive in toothpaste. As I already mentioned, the sand in toothpaste can cause tooth wear with too much brushing.

**Sorbitol and saccharin** are both sweeteners and are used in toothpaste. They are on the list of substances we want to avoid.

**Titanium dioxide** is a pigment used for providing brightness and whiteness. It is used as a stain remover and a whitener. Titanium dioxide is potentially carcinogenic in humans.[254] If the titanium dioxide in toothpaste contained nano-sized particles then it can be toxic to cells in your body and absorb through contact.[255]

**Glycerin** is added to toothpaste to give it its "pasty" consistency and helps prevent the toothpaste from drying out. Supposedly, glycerin requires 27 rinses to remove from the teeth. This glycerin film could create a barrier on the teeth that would prevent teeth from getting harder and stronger. Usually, small amounts of toothpaste get swallowed or absorbed directly into your bloodstream through your gums through a process called diffusion.

**Sodium Lauryl Sulfate** is used as a foaming agent and a degreaser. It is used also for washing cars and cleaning garage floors. It is absorbed by the body and can damage or affect cells. It has been correlated with canker sores.

## *Natural Tooth Cleaners*

1. Sea salt. Just dab a small amount on your tooth brush.

2. Homemade tooth powder (recipe provided).

3. Herbal tooth powders (one recipe provided).

4. Toothsoap. A liquid soap made with coconut, olive and palm oils. It makes tooth brushing fun. You can purchase it at **www.mytoothsoap. com** and the coupon code SMILE will give you an extra discount!

5. Orappeal System is available at: **naturalief.com**

6. Any type of natural cleaning agent that uses herbs or liquids that has no chemicals or ingredients on the label you cannot pronounce or grow in a garden.

# Tooth Brushing

As we learned from Dr. Phillips in the gum disease chapter, tooth brushing can be fine for teeth if the bristles are soft and if there is not too much abrasion, but it can rapidly wear away your gums and even cause gum disease. This is because brushing pushes the plaque into the gingival sulcus where the gums meet the teeth. For tooth brushing to be healthy, you need to use blotting or at least an oral irrigator after brushing to remove the plaque at the gum line.

Soft tooth brushes with rounded ends help avoid eroding tooth enamel. Electric brushes which have an electromagnetic component to them do a superior job of cleaning but they may lead to some minor EMF exposure. There is also risk with electric toothbrushes of damaging the gums because of the high speed of the vibrations. If you use one, be careful.

# Tooth and Gum Healing

While tooth liquid products clean the teeth, products made with herbs can heal the teeth and gums in a different way. Herbs can build, pull out toxins, and nourish. Herbal tooth powder can be found at some health food stores—make sure they do not have any toxic additives. Good herbal tooth and gum mixtures are *Tooth and Gum Restore Formula* by Dr. Richard Schulze (this can be used with an oral irrigator) and *Dr. Christopher's Herbal Tooth & Gum Powder.* I encourage you to try a few different tooth-cleaning products and locate one that feels good to you. You can also make your own toothpowder at home.

**Peppermint Tooth Powder Recipe**

> 2 tablespoons baking soda (pure sodium bicarbonate only)

> 1 teaspoon finely ground sea salt

> 5–10 drops of organic peppermint essential oil (available in natural food stores or online)

**Baking Soda and Gums**
Baking soda alkalizes the mouth. When the mouth is too acidic then tooth decay can be present. When the mouth is too alkaline, then this might contribute to gum disease. I have had mixed reports on baking soda and gums. Some reports say baking soda irritates the gums. Others have healed tooth abscesses with baking soda.

**Herbal Tooth and Gum Powder Recipe**
The following recipe makes a fabulous tooth powder. I purchase herbs at the local herb shop and grind them in a coffee grinder. The recipe is from the late master herbalist Dr. John Christopher.

> 3 parts oak bark

> 6 parts comfrey root

> 3 parts horsetail grass

> 1 part lobelia

> 1 part cloves

> 3 parts peppermint

People need to be aware of the herbs they use, and use them wisely. (With prolonged and exclusive use, this tooth powder may cause some slight tooth discoloration that can be cleaned off.) I alternate using this herbal formula with the baking soda formula. The tooth and gum powder can also be placed on gums for gum healing.

## Flossing

Flossing is literally a double-edged sword. Since many of us do not have perfectly aligned teeth, food can get caught in between teeth. The disadvantage to flossing is that it is very easy to cut your gums. Injuring your gums daily does not seem like a practice that will promote healthy teeth and gums. The advantage to flossing is that you are able to clean out debris from between your teeth that would otherwise linger and putrefy in your mouth.

If you floss your teeth, be very careful not to slash your gums. Using dental tape, which is a wide and thick version of dental floss, is the recommended flossing technique of tooth hygiene specialist dentist Robert. O. Nara. There is evidence from Dr. Phillips that flossing with string is not a part of good dental health. Using the blotting method to poke out food with an ultrasoft tooth brush, or using a water flosser (oral irrigator) seems to be much better suggestions. If you choose to floss with a string, then use dental tape.

# *The Fluoride Deception*

**Fluoride does not heal tooth cavities**. There are different forms of fluoride, and the one put in drinking water is usually hydrofluosilicic acid. In 1986–1987, a study involving 39,207 children aged 5–17 showed no statistical difference in tooth decay from using non-fluoridated or fluoridated water.[256] Several large scale studies worldwide show the same results.[257] According to data published in the July 2009 *Journal of the American Dental Association* children's cavity rates are similar whether the water is fluoridated or not.[258]

**Fluoride is dangerous**. Most of the fluoride used in water supplies is toxic waste from the fertilizer industry.[259] The Environmental Protection Agency's Employee Union (consisting of approximately 1500 scientists, lawyers, engineers and other professional employees) is opposed to water fluoridation. The EPA Union states:

> *Scientific literature documents the increasingly out-of-control exposures to fluoride, the lack of benefit to dental health from ingestion of fluoride and the hazards to human health from such ingestion.*[260]

Fluoride is an enzyme and hormone inhibitor, affecting the nervous system as well as digestion. Fluoride is the major cause of brittle bones and teeth, and is responsible for causing mottled enamel, producing white, light gray or brown spots on the teeth. Fluoride actually alters the natural biological creation of tooth enamel and creates false, more brittle tooth enamel (which now contains fluorapatite). This false enamel is no better at preventing tooth decay than regular tooth enamel in the long term. A stronger barrier to bacteria is not what keeps tooth decay at bay, but rather a balanced internal body chemistry from good food habits.

Fluoride may cause brain and kidney damage, a decrease in I.Q., and may cross the placental barrier in pregnant women. Water fluoridation has also been linked to cancer. In 1977 Dr. Dean Burk, former chief chemist of the US National Cancer Institute, and Dr. John Yiamouyiannis, president of the Safe Water Foundation proved that water fluoridation increased the risk of cancer. Their studies concluded that:

*One-tenth of the 350,000 cancer deaths per year in the U.S. are linked with artificial public water fluoridation.[261]*

The U.S. Congress called for animal studies to confirm these results and the studies were released in 1990. The studies showed clear evidence that fluoride does cause cancer.[262]

A majority of Europe does not use water fluoridation and neither should we. Countries that rejected fluoridation on the grounds that its use is unethical and that it imposes unnecessary health risks include: Austria, Belgium, Denmark, Finland, France, Germany, Holland, Hungary, Italy, Iceland, Luxembourg, Netherlands, Norway, Sweden and Yugoslavia.

Nature has given us the map for perfect tooth enamel, impervious to tooth decay. We can maintain a high immunity to tooth decay without fluoride, provided we obey Nature's laws, eat a proper diet rich in calcium, phosphorus, and the fat-soluble vitamins, and avoid overly processed nutrient-devoid foods. Synthetically derived fluoride cannot replace or reproduce the total harmony of Nature's design.

I do not recommend that you drink fluoridated water or use fluoridated toothpaste. Do not submit to dental treatments that contain fluoride. Because of fluoride's damaging effects on the glandular system, it is possible to get weak enamel from fluoride, so check with your local water board to find out if your water supply is fluoridated. If it is, then you need to purchase a special fluoride filter or have fluoride free water delivered to you.

Placing fluoride in toothpaste and into our water supply is a crime. It is unethical because fluoride has never been proven safe and effective. In fact, the opposite has been proven to be true. I urge you to support efforts to eradicate fluoride use in the United States. Please visit the Fluoride Action Network, **fluoridealert.org**, and The Fluoride Education Project, **poisonfluoride.com/pfpc**.

## Tooth Decay is Not an Infectious Disease

I have shown how it is now scientifically proven that bacteria are not the main cause of cavities by the life's work of dentist Ralph Steinman in explaining the dentinal fluid transport mechanism. When dentist Percy Howe tried to inoculate bacteria into guinea pigs to cause tooth decay or gum disease, he could not. He could only cause cavities with a change in diet. The bacterial theory of cavities is justified through the assertion that tooth decay is an infectious disease. This infectious disease theory is false for several reasons:

1. Antibiotics that kill bacteria do not stop tooth decay.

2. People do not develop antibodies to tooth decay.

3. Antibacterial mouth rinses do not effectively prevent cavities.

4. Once you are infected with tooth decay you do not develop immunity
to it unless your diet is dramatically improved.

Bacteria exist symbiotically in our mouths at all times and evolve and change as
our health does. Hence, no antibacterial remedy will ever cure tooth decay.

# Moving Beyond Painful Dentistry

The truth remains that a significant majority of dental treatments are unnecessary when diet is changed and teeth remineralize as they are biologically designed
to do. The big question that remains unanswered is why haven't we been told
the truth about our teeth from modern dentistry? Weston Price's research with
indigenous diets was published many decades ago in the *Journal of the American
Dental Association*, so his treatment successes and research findings were widely
available.

In this chapter we have looked at the high price we have paid for modern
dentistry. Modern dentistry is an unequivocal failure. Treatments from conventional dentists are highly toxic and usually disease-promoting such as fluoride,
mercury fillings, leaky root canals and metal tooth fillings. Holistic and biological
dentists offer more natural, less toxic alternatives to modern dentistry. This is a
huge improvement, but few of them offer the real cure, which is found through
diet and the balancing of body chemistry.

I am not trying to destroy the dental profession. The dental profession is
destructive, and is destroying itself. What I ask of the dental profession is for it
to change and evolve. The future of dentistry lies in disease prevention through
proper nutrition and body chemistry balancing, along with minimally invasive
methods to correct dental arch problems and bite problems. Imagine being able
to find a cavity before it happens, and then remineralize it with nutritional intervention? We have the ability and the technology to do this today; we simply lack
the desire, care, willingness, and legal framework to provide this level of treatment to the public. This would be real dentistry: finding and preventing cavities
completely organically before tooth enamel was lost, and before tooth infections
occurred. Dentists could still earn very decent livings by analyzing blood chemistry, examining teeth, offering nutritional consulting, and repairing bite imbalances non-surgically. As long as a dentist's income is tied to performing invasive
treatments, where more severe treatments mean greater profit, the current state
of modern dentistry will remain a rotten profession.

Making dentistry work for all of us means changing the rules of the profession. The dentist of the future will not be focused on performing complex tooth
surgery. This will be a specialty field. All a preventative dentist would need to
know is how to check for cavities and how to help people intervene with their diet
using the most modern and scientifically proven methods (such as fermented cod

liver oil) and they will cure a large portion of people's cavities before they even happen. Imagine seeing a DPD, a doctor of preventative dentistry, or a DDH, a doctor of dental health, who would help you keep your teeth healthy and strong naturally with diet, supplements, herbs and homeopathy.

A large percentage of our population is suffering from poor health, physical stress, and a loss of vitality from bite disorders. There is a vast and largely untapped market for holistic methods to return the upper and lower jaw to their harmonious state and bring balance to the facial structures while healing head, neck and jaw pain. This will make people happier, more relaxed, and more resistant to disease.

The problem with modern dentistry is that to become a licensed dentist, you must spend most of your schooling learning how to perform dental surgery. Yet what really matters in this new school of truly holistic dentistry that I propose in this book is preventing tooth decay and repairing the bite with non-surgical and holistic methods. Yet these methods are not currently being taught to dentists in dental school. The training in dental school does not give dentists the foundation needed to be effective nutrition counselors and efficient bite repairers. Furthermore there needs to be more of an integrative care model which emphasizes the health of the entire body so that the art and science of dentistry can complement and work synergistically with all the other health professions.

There is no longer any reason for the population at large to be afflicted with tooth decay (dental caries). Join me now in voicing an urgent call to change the way we administer oral health in our country. "Dentistry, we need you to change!"

*Chapter 9*

# Your Bite:
# A Hidden Cause of Cavities

## *A Fresh Look at Orthodontics and TMJ*

I want to introduce you to an extraordinary world that is literally right under your nose: your bite. Your bite has a substantial relationship to your overall health, your strength, your vitality, your level of attractiveness as well as your susceptibility to tooth decay. Super athletes know these facts and regularly wear mouth guards such as the Pure Power Mouthguard™ which slides the jaw into a more correct muscular and skeletal position. These adjustments increase overall muscle strength and endurance.

In this chapter you will discover the reasons for temporomandibular joint (TMJ) dysfunction, a deeper understanding of the mechanics of orthodontics and braces, and the important connections between the position of your bite to tooth decay and your overall health. Best of all, you will discover how to improve your health through correcting the position of your bite. Theories about the treatment and alignment of the bite are often obscured by contention, closed-mindedness and limited vision. Therefore be prepared to be met with that attitude from many practitioners in the field if you bring them information that is beyond the realm of their belief systems, such as what I will present here.

## *Your Ideal Jaw Position and Enjoyment of Life*

To understand how our jaw and skull are supposed to be aligned, let us look at examples of ideal physical development as our template. Native peoples across the globe who displayed immunity to tooth decay also possessed what Weston Price called "splendidly formed dental arches."[263] The dental arch is comprised of the maxilla, the upper palate of the mouth, and the mandible, the jaw bone. In general, the better the nutrition of the individual throughout life, beginning from before conception, the wider the dental arches (the upper and lower jaws) will be. Wider arches mean wider, rounder faces that we subconsciously associate with both robust health and natural attractiveness. These qualities can influence how one chooses a partner who will likely be a successful mother with excellent reproductive capacities, since generally a wide dental arch indicates the pelvic

## Ancient Skulls Reveal Perfect Occlusion

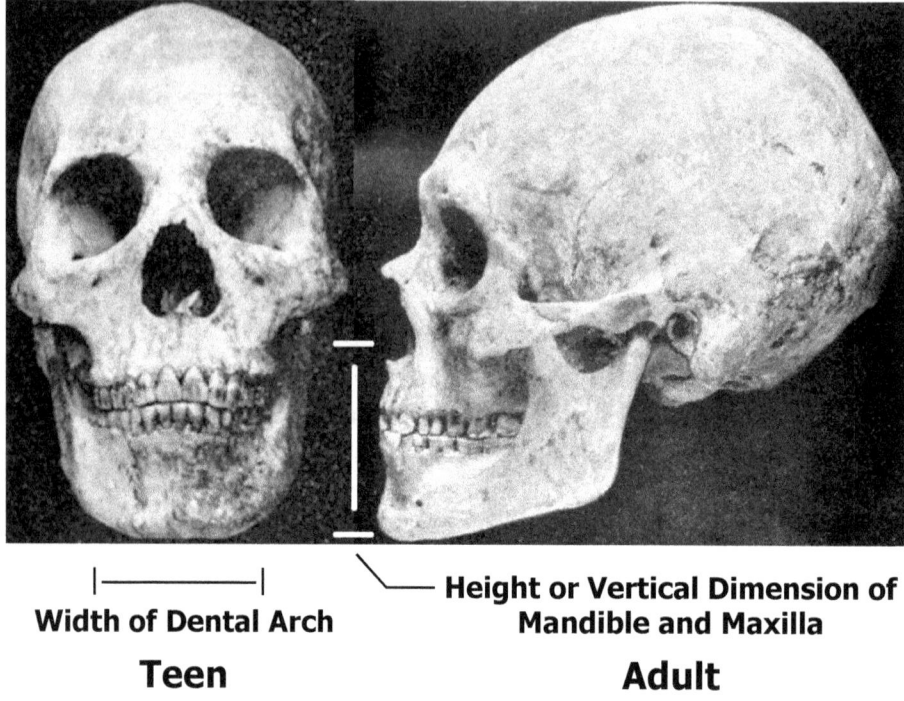

|————————|            ╲———— **Height or Vertical Dimension of**
**Width of Dental Arch**                    **Mandible and Maxilla**

## Teen                                    Adult

brim will also be spacious enough to ensure easier births. I describe this in more detail in my book about preconception, pregnancy, parenting, and children's health called *Healing Our Children.* You can learn more about it as well as obtain the book at **www.healingourchildren.org**

When you look at this photo of two human skulls, you may assume that they are simply ordinary human skulls and you do not see anything of interest. What I want you to look at carefully in these skulls is how the teeth of the maxilla and mandible line up. The top front teeth and the bottom front teeth are flush with each other and line up "tip to tip." There is no overbite and there is no underbite. All of the teeth appear to be in contact with one another. Although not visible in the pictures, in an ideal bite there ought to be a paper-thin gap in the front teeth so they do not put pressure upon each other in the relaxed jaw position. These skulls show us our therapeutic model for natural human development. Most of us do not have bites that fit in this position when our mouths are closed. This is not so because of a genetic predisposition, but because a poor diet and other nutritional or environmental toxins have prevented a majority of the population from having fully formed maxillas (upper palates) and mandibles (lower jaws).

# Genetics versus Intercepted Heredity

Tooth decay is not a genetic condition. It is a factor of the environment, and usually the primary environmental factor is poor nutrition. When nature cannot fulfill its ideal potential, we have a situation called blocked or intercepted heredity. Crooked teeth and wisdom teeth that do not fit (as well as over- and underbites) **are not genetic traits**. These problems occur from the lack of proper nutritional building blocks. Further documentation of this fact is available in Weston Price's book, *Nutrition and Physical Degeneration*. When our bodies lack the proper ingredients for building bones or there is an alteration in the metabolism of calcium and phosphorous, our bodies will not be perfectly formed to fulfill our hereditary potential. The structure and mineralization of our jaws and teeth suffer as a result of deficiencies in our modern nutritional program. This is similar to the growth of a plant in unfertile soil. The plant will not blossom to its full potential. To grow healthy teeth and bones requires whole and unrefined foods carefully grown and prepared, and a diet high in fat-soluble vitamins and phosphorus. Weston Price explains how the Aborigines of Australia had perfectly developed jaws for untold generations until they changed their diet.

> It is most remarkable and should be one of the most challenging facts that can come to our modern civilization that such primitive races as the Aborigines of Australia have reproduced for generation after generation through many centuries — no one knows for how many thousands of years — without the development of a conspicuous number of irregularities of the dental arches. Yet, in the next generation after these people adopt the foods of the white man, a large percentage of the children developed irregularities of the dental arches with conspicuous facial deformities. The deformity patterns are similar to those seen in white civilizations. [264]

# Why Teeth are Crowded and Wisdom Teeth are Misaligned

When physical development is impeded primarily by a poor and deficient diet, Nature's blueprint of a fully developed maxilla (palate) and mandible (jaw) remains incomplete. As a result the maxilla and mandible are not as wide as they need to be and there is not enough space for all of the teeth. When the teeth come in, they appear crowded. Therefore, there is no such thing as teeth that are too big, but rather it is a jaw that is too small. This condition also makes wisdom teeth come in crooked, or causes the roots of wisdom teeth to be impacted.

## Healthy Bite and Misaligned Bite

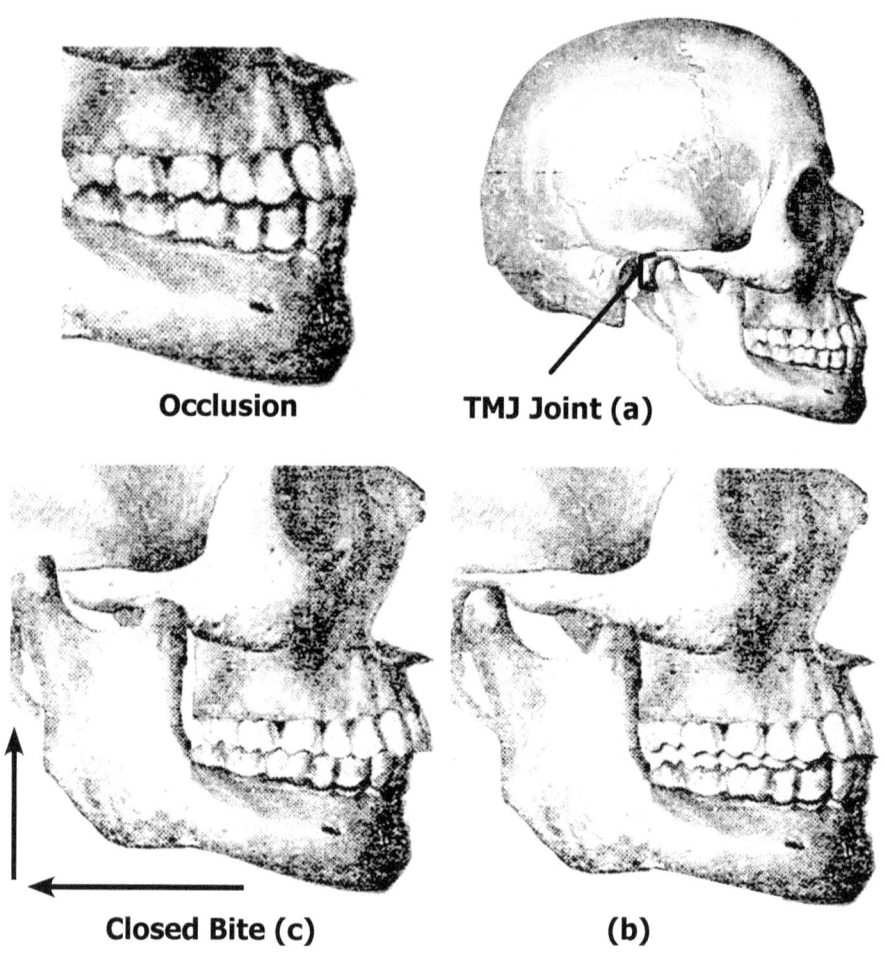

**Occlusion**    **TMJ Joint (a)**

**Closed Bite (c)**    **(b)**

. . . . . . . . . . . . . . . . . . . . . . . . . . . . . . . . . . . . . . . . . . . . . . . . . . . . . . . . . . .

Occlusion:
Occlusion is how our teeth come together when we chew and when our mouth is at rest.

. . . . . . . . . . . . . . . . . . . . . . . . . . . . . . . . . . . . . . . . . . . . . . . . . . . . . . . . . . .

# *Your Bite and TMJ Pain, Night Grinding, and Tooth Decay*

The trigeminal nerve is the largest nerve in your head. It has a network of fibers that run throughout your face in an intricate matrix. The trigeminal nerve has three major branches: the mandibular (jaw) nerve, the maxillary (upper palate) nerve, and the ophthalmic (eye) nerve. The trigeminal nerve system fans throughout your entire face, and contains pain, position and movement (sensory and motor) sensors and control mechanisms. The nerves of each tooth are connected to either the manidibular or maxillary branch of the trigeminal nerve. When you have a toothache, the nerve pain goes right through the trigeminal nerve and communicates directly to your thalamus and cerebral cortex. This explains why you feel tooth pain so very intensely. The trigeminal nerve connects with our limbic brain which is related to emotions and mental functions.[265] How you bite is directly connected with how you feel.

When your mouth closes, your jaw should be in a relaxed and comfortable position. The correct positioning of the jaw and teeth is shown in both figure *a* and in the figure labeled *occlusion*. In figure *a*, the molars naturally and comfortably touch on all surfaces when the jaw is in the closed, relaxed position. When the back molars are touching comfortably, the body's nervous system is sent a constant signal of relaxation through the trigeminal nerve. Because of this nerve relaxation, a person with contacting molars in the comfortable, relaxed position ages more slowly, heals faster, has a positive outlook on life, and generally feels good.

Take a moment and look in the mirror. You can see if your jaw is naturally in position *a*. If it is not, do not be surprised, as 95% or more of the population has a misaligned jaw. The term for a misaligned bite is *malocclusion*. When your jaw is misaligned the sensory system of the trigeminal nerve is activated.[266] A classic jaw misalignment is called a *closed bite*. When the jaw hinges closed through its natural motion as in figure *b*, the molars do not touch. Rather the front teeth collide into one another. This unfortunate circumstance resulted because the jaw bone did not develop to its full potential, and the back molars are too low. Because either the upper back molars or lower ones did not extend to their fullest potential, the jaw cannot relax in the neutral closed position as demonstrated in figure *a*.

A closed and relaxed jaw as shown in the skull photographs and in figure *a* is especially important during sleep. The body regenerates while we sleep. But if the molars are not comfortably touching, as in figure *b*, then side effects such as night time tooth grinding or clenching can occur. As the teeth clench at night, if they are in positions *b* or *c* they can easily become worn down and overly stressed since the molars are not comfortably supporting the mouth. This is exactly why teeth become infected and eroded. This situation can also be associated with snoring and loss of fully restful sleep.

What also happens in the condition illustrated by figure *b* is the body's sensory nervous system receives messages through the trigeminal nerve to the brain that the jaw is not relaxed. The body then tries to make the molars contact one another to find the relaxed and natural position. Yet in order for the body to find a natural biting position and for the molars to touch as they were designed to, the jaw must hinge backwards and upwards as shown in figure *c*. Since the body seeks relaxation, and since chewing and eating require the front teeth to avoid colliding while the molars grind food, what happens is that the jaw must hinge in a forced manner to compensate. While the jaw joint is capable of sliding forward and backward, it is not supposed to slide backward all the time. In figure *c* you see the final *closed bite* position; the molars are touching now, but the jaw is jammed backwards. At the same time, the front teeth may be contacting each other wrongly and wearing down. Over time, the hinging of the jaw in the unnatural position overly strains the thin friction disk in the temporomandibular joint, and there is pain, popping, and cracking on the light end of the symptom scale. The worst thing about this common condition is that the body rarely or never is able to completely relax, heal and regenerate. Instead there is a constant experience of tension.

· · · · · · · · · · · · · · · · · · · · · · · · · · · · · · · · · · · · · · · · · · · · · · · · · · ·

### Electro-Magnetic Fields (EMF) and Cavities

Some people experience tooth pain when exposed to electro-magnetic fields such as from a television or a computer monitor. The connection between our nervous system and our teeth could explain why this happens.

· · · · · · · · · · · · · · · · · · · · · · · · · · · · · · · · · · · · · · · · · · · · · · · · · · ·

## Root Canals, Tooth Infections and Your Bite

A significant proportion of tooth infections have at their source a usually unrecognized component of bite dysfunction. Nighttime clenching and daytime stress from the molars not comfortably touching cause strain on specific teeth depending on how the jaw is misaligned. Nighttime clenching is also one of the main causes of abfractions—gum line ridges and sensitivity of teeth caused by relentless stresses from the jaw pressures that wear them down.

When the jaw cannot comfortably close as in figures *b* and *c* then certain teeth can become severely worn or traumatized. The body has a hard time healing those specific teeth because they are constantly being bruised, and these are the exact teeth that become painful and infected. A poor bite is one of the main reasons why people develop tooth infections.

## The "Feel Good" Substance P

Neuropeptides are a type of molecule our nervous system uses to communicate. *Substance P* is a neuropeptide that stimulates inflammation and also functions in the transmission of pain signals within the nervous system. So when you have a toothache, there is a marked increase in substance P. If you have an injury in your body, amounts of substance P increase near the injury site. After substance P is released from your nerves it lingers in your body for a while.[267]

The trigeminal nerve has such a high density of pain fibers that it can have a dramatic effect on the substance P levels in your body. Substance P is actually good for us. It stimulates cell growth and promotes wound healing.[268] But when someone's bite is out of alignment such as shown in figure *c* then the trigeminal nerve which is laced throughout the mandible (jaw) releases pain signals through substance P in large amounts. Perhaps this happens because the body correlates the jaw misalignment with a physical injury. The constant release of substance P from the trigeminal nerve over time causes our sensory system to become over stimulated or hyperactive. This then substantially reduces our body's ability to send substance P to the parts of our body that require healing and regeneration. Therefore when our bite is out of alignment we heal more slowly. Too much substance P in the system leads to a burned out nervous system. It can cause hyperactivity in children. Excess substance P from bite imbalances leads to hyper-sensitivity to touch, smells, light, and loud noises as well as to general irritabil-ity.[269] Disease conditions that respond well to jaw alignment include fibromyalgia, irritable bowel syndrome, autism, asthma, and all of the autoimmune disorders.

When your jaw is relaxed, then substance P is not being overly released because your jaw is aligned. Substance P then can do its job to help heal and regenerate all the parts of your body. A relaxed jaw from a correct bite makes your body relaxed and your body rejuvenates itself. A relaxed bite keeps us youth-ful, helps us heal well, and have strength and energy when we need it. This is the power of your bite.

## *Your Bite and Your Vitality*

The excess of substance P released from a bad bite in part explains why neuro-logical and physical function usually improve dramatically when the jaw is in the relaxed and neutral position as seen in figure *a*. Mouth guards that improve the strength and vitality of athletes move the jaw into a more biologically cor-rect position. The body senses through the trigeminal nerve that everything is in alignment, the nervous system relaxes, and the body functions more optimally.[270] As a result, strength, endurance, and reaction times increase. There are early stud-ies that indicate that jaw clenching and chewing have an anti-stress effect and are stress coping mechanisms, provided the bite is correct.[271]

## *How TMJ and Bite Affect Cavities,*
## *Tooth Infections and Toothaches*

When your bite is out of alignment, your body receives pain signals via substance P. A misaligned bite affects cavities and tooth pain in three ways. First, the nervous system of the jaw is hyper stimulated which inhibits the natural healing response of the body to mend damaged teeth. Second, when the bite is out of balance, specific teeth become overly stressed from the mechanical forces of the jaw. Third, with a bad bite, the trigeminal nerve becomes hypersensitive. With these conditions a toothache will hurt much more than it normally should. What this means for you is that if you have a tooth ache, or tooth infection, then any types of body therapy you can do to relax the stresses on your nervous system, particularly the trigeminal nerve, can dramatically impact the health of your teeth. Perhaps half or more of tooth infections and tooth pain can be healed simply by helping the jaw relax and by moving the bite into a more correct position.

## Profound Effects of TMJ Dysfunction and a Bad Bite

TMJ dysfunction (TMD) can present symptoms such as pain behind eyes, difficulty opening and closing the mouth, ringing in ears, tooth grinding, over clenching, worn teeth, headaches and even vision problems. If the jaw is allowed to hinge normally and does not need to be forced into the closed bite position as shown in figure *c* then the TMD symptoms can resolve if the joint is not excessively damaged. The method of resolution of TMD is usually some type of dental appliance which helps the jaw function correctly.

Pain with TMD is caused by overwork of the nervous and muscular systems as they must function in an unnatural manner to bring the teeth together for chewing and the natural jaw clenching position. Over time the muscles fatigue, become strained, and can lead to pain in the jaw, the back of the neck, head and ears.[272]

The hyper stimulated nervous system has some surprising side effects. For example, orthopedic orthodontist Dr. Brendan Stack believes that the basis of most of the symptoms of Tourette's syndrome is essentially a misalignment of the mandible to the base of the skull. By correcting the position of the jaw with a dental appliance, the eye blinking, eyelid tics, mouth tics, head nodding, shoulder shrugging and head tremors disappear. Dr. Stack has videos on his website that appear to depict miracles. Yet the amazing recoveries are based on a correct understanding of how the jaw and cranial system were meant to function. You can see immobilized people walking again within minutes at **www.tmjstack.com**

Many diseases, particularly neurological diseases like autism, have a significant symptom component in that the bite of the afflicted individual is severely compromised. Symptoms of a severely misaligned bite are a crooked face, improper facial growth, the mouth hanging open, tongue sticking out, and a very poor posture. Not all bite misalignments are that obvious. An imbalance of as little as $1/8$ of an inch can cause malocclusion and health problems.[273] Treating and resolving diseases that have nervous system components can require a therapeutic correction of the bite. Unfortunately the connection between neurological diseases and the bite is often completely overlooked.

# Orthodontics

Now we will learn why braces are generally unnecessary and in fact harmful. First, two definitions:

> **Orthodontics** is the practice of forcing teeth to appear to be in alignment using non-removable dental appliances such as braces.

> **Dental Orthopedics** is a medical model that focuses on the structure and alignment of the cranial bones, with the intent to align the jaw towards its normal developmental state. "Functional orthodontics" is another name for this modality.

Many people have chosen orthodontics, which is a means of making their teeth to appear straight, when they really wanted orthopedics, which is the correction of physical development to a normal and healthy state. These terms lead to a great deal of confusion because there are conventional orthodontists, orthodontist-orthopedists, and dental orthopedists. For clarity I will refer to practitioners who only look at making teeth straight, and who take a mechanistic approach that works against the normal function of the body as conventional orthodontists. Orthopedists are dental practitioners who align the bite, even though some orthopedists may also call themselves orthodontists.

Dental orthopedics is the art form of reconstructing bites with dental appliances. This entails more than merely a mechanical process, but involves an artistic non-surgical cranial reconstruction. Conventional orthodontics is a mechanistic system that does not consider the normal developmental model of the body.

I, like many others, have experienced negative outcomes from conventional orthodontics. When I was young, my jaw was in the position as shown in figure *c,* also referred to as an overbite. Because the goal of conventional orthodontists (who practice orthodontics, not orthopedics) is to make teeth straight, without even necessarily making them contact properly, their simplified approach is to make your teeth straight BY ANY MEANS NECCESSARY. The conventional orthodontist believes that the jaws are stuck in one position and cannot move. At best, all an orthodontist sees is what is shown in the figure labeled *occlusion:* a row of teeth. The orthodontist, like the conventional dentist, also sees a row of money. I remember my orthodontist had nice pictures on his office wall of his mansion, and of his family's many vacations to Hawaii. The conventional orthodontic approach was designed as a business model and is an easy and convenient way to move through many patients in an assembly-line fashion. In the process, the conventional orthodontist rakes in large profits while ignorantly thwarting the normal developmental processes of the body.

In order to make the teeth straight and my jaw look a certain way (or to get my teeth to touch in a certain way; the goal was never made clear to me), by any means necessary, I was required to wear a headgear. The theory (wrongly) goes that when children are growing (I was eight) pushing the maxilla (upper palate) against its natural growth direction with a tortuous device called a headgear that is worn nightly, will cause the mandible (the jaw) to catch up. And then the hope is that the teeth will touch correctly (occlusion). So the fairytale goes, and everyone will be happy, and the orthodontist will get his $5,000.

Fifteen years later, however, at the age of 23, my teeth did not touch at all naturally. I developed TMJ dysfunction (TMD) by the time I was 30 years old, my lower teeth became very crooked, and my jaw never moved forward the way it was supposed to according to the treatment protocol. The conventional orthodontist's model of arresting the development of the maxilla is misguided since the body rarely or never overgrows a part of itself, rather other parts of the body do not grow fully so the maxilla appears to protrude, but it is really normal.

The results of two years of torture for me as a child were a lot of money spent, but no positive outcome. I know many other people who have gone through similar treatment, and have similar TMD and other serious problems to show for it. The problems get worse over time because our jaw continues to grow, or imbalances get worse, meanwhile the TMJ joint wears out. Many people do not figure out that they have TMD until, sadly, the entire joint is nearly worn out. I am lucky in a way. I have spent so much time researching dental problems that my research kept me focusing on my bite, and I finally realized my body was in a constant state of stress because my molars did not touch properly. Don't worry if this sounds like your situation; I will explain how to treat this problem shortly.

## Dental Orthopedics Focuses on Normal Development

Conventional orthodontics pursues the wrong goal, which is to make teeth straight BY ANY MEANS NECESSARY. However, to create a healthy bite, the jaw and cranium must be aligned in natural position and size. This is the goal of dental orthopedics. If you have a closed bite as illustrated in figure c, the orthopedic treatment might include insertion of a dental appliance which has a plastic spacer that sits on top of the molars, such as a twin block or an OmNi-2. This is seen in the figure where the bite height is restored with a plastic spacer. This allows the jaw to stay comfortably closed in a natural position even though the molars do not naturally touch. What is amazing about the use of such an appliance is that when there is a space such that certain molars do not touch, the molars start to get closer together as the jaw bone grows in under the molars. Eventually over

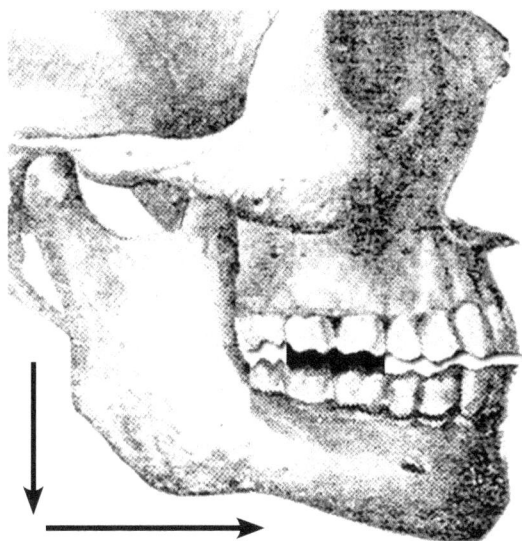

**Bite Height Restored**

a treatment period of eighteen months to three years all of the molars can be guided to meet each other, and the correct functional bite height can be retained without further need of a dental appliance.

## *Conventional Orthodontic Practices Damage Faces*

Conventional orthodontic practices damage facial aesthetics.[274] They also damage the functionality of the bite as seen in many cases of TMD from just a small informal survey of people who have undergone conventional orthodontic treatment. The most damaging aspects of orthodontics are tooth extractions and head gear.

Many patients or parents are not adequately informed about the dangers of conventional orthodontics prior to treatment.[275] In particular the resorption of tooth roots is a common and sometimes highly damaging result of wearing braces. Root resorption is the loss or damage to the tooth root from the pulling force of braces. When you move teeth with braces, a tooth does not simply slide into the next position. The figure of the tooth in chapter three shows how the tooth is surrounded by bone. To move a tooth, the braces pull the teeth and the tooth is pushed into the alveolar bone. This is something akin to a boat traveling through thick ice. As the tooth is pushed in one direction, the bone in the jaw must dissolve on one end of the tooth and fill in on the other side of the tooth for the tooth to move. When the tooth roots are pushed against the jaw bone with fixed dental appliances like braces, 93% of them are damaged; some severely.[276] Approximately 72-84% of teeth that have been treated with a fixed appliance (braces) have suffered clinically significant damage.[277] As a result many teeth suffer permanent damage from braces. Gum disease later in life, in combination with roots that are damaged from braces and are therefore much shorter, means early tooth loss. Standard consent and disclaimer forms that patients must sign before accepting braces as treatment explain the known harm caused by braces. They include jaw pain (from the bite being pulled out of alignment), root resorption, tooth or jaw instability, fleeting results due to physical growth, gum inflammation, and unexpected results. Meanwhile, in the orthopedic model you will suffer none of these side effects because the dental orthopedic model works with the natural form of the body, helping it function and grow properly.

If you put braces on the teeth of a growing child, and do not even try to move or push teeth, as the child's jaw grows, his teeth are going to move in the jaw bone. Root resorption is worse in older children than in younger children.[278]

• • • • • • • • • • • • • • • • • • • • • • • • • • • • • • • • • • • • • • • • • • •

**Bicuspid Extraction**
Bicuspid extraction performed by conventional orthodontics on children and teens collapses the structure of the face, making the face more narrow and less attractive. This unfortunate result has been shown in studies comparing differing orthodontic approaches with identical twins. Over time, the twin whose teeth were not extracted, but whose dental arch was widened instead, developed the more attractive facial features. Bicuspid extraction sacrifices perfectly healthy and beautiful teeth to the faulty goals of conventional orthodontics.[279] Not to mention the fact that pulling teeth can cause emotional trauma as children feel that they have been disfigured or that there is something wrong with them.

• • • • • • • • • • • • • • • • • • • • • • • • • • • • • • • • • • • • • • • • • • •

# Orthodontics Does Not Address the Physiological Cause of Crooked Teeth

Crooked teeth are the result of a maxilla (upper palate) that is too narrow.[280] This leads to a child having a more narrow face and less appealing looks. Practically speaking a wider face means more space for the tongue, and a greater ease in breathing, along with plenty of space for all of the teeth including the wisdom teeth. What conventional orthodontics does is make space for teeth by pushing the teeth, rather than by encouraging the jaw to develop to its full potential, which is the orthopedic approach. In their drive to make teeth fit, conventional orthodontists pull out teeth. Yet extracting teeth has led to noticeably altered facial features to the patient's detriment. [281] The other conventional method for making all of the teeth fit besides extractions is to fan them out forward. Part of the problem with the bite in an individual with an overbite (closed bite), is not enough height in the molars for the jaw to swing forward naturally and to have the molars comfortably touch. When the teeth are fanned out with braces, the back molars stay at the same low height, and then the height of the front teeth is also lowered by being rocked outward.

Rather than working with the correct therapeutic model as described earlier and the natural growth direction of the body, conventional orthodontics works against it. Rather than bringing the jaw forward, conventional orthodontics pushes the maxilla (upper palate) back and compounds the problem and further prevents the mandible (jaw) from growing.[282] Conventional orthodontics lowers the height of teeth that do not need to be lowered, removes teeth that are perfectly beautiful and healthy, pushes teeth into the jaw bone and causes their roots to shorten. **To say that conventional orthodontics is a massive disaster would be a grave understatement.**

The wires in orthodontic appliances contain nickel and can cause personality changes such as a lack of affection and lowered intelligence. Homeopathic remedies for nickel poisoning can resolve this situation.

## Functional Orthopedics

The good news is that nearly every problem with orthodontics can be corrected to some degree with orthopedics. Finding a practitioner who understands all of the aspects and integrative care required for dental orthopedic changes can be difficult since dental orthopedics requires the specialty of three or more areas of expertise. As a result, the combination of a dentist who practices orthopedics along with physical therapies is required for the best treatment outcomes. Dental orthopedics requires not just an understanding of, but the physical manipulation of the cranial bones, the jaw bones, the TMJ joint, the fascia which is a fibrous tissue that surrounds muscles, nerves, and the *dura mater* which surrounds the brain and spinal cord. The younger the patient, and the less severe the imbalance, the less expertise is going to be required from multiple fields to produce a successful result.

### Craniopathy

Craniopathy has its origins in an old system of chiropractic work. When we breathe, the bones in our head actually breathe and expand. The human head contains a set of 23 interlocking bones. There are eight cranial bones and fourteen facial bones. When we are born, many of us have slight imbalances in the bones of our body, particularly the cranial bones. This creates a cranial birth distortion. Over time these distortions, or bone malformations in the cranium or cervical vertebrae, can lead to bite distortions, particularly left/right imbalances where one side of the jaw develops more fully than the other. Injuries and other traumas in life can also cause cranial bones to become stuck, which over time can cause physiological problems.

The other important understanding with relation to braces or any functional orthopedic appliance therapy is that every time you move even one tooth, some or all of the 23 cranial bones are going to move with it. This is because the tooth is attached to our jaw bone. The *dura mater* and fascia also move when teeth are moved.

The net result of the interconnection of cranial bones and teeth is that it is possible to go through an entire round of orthopedics or orthodontics and have the jaw and bite function perfectly, but still have a distorted cranial system. If the distorted cranial system in that situation is fixed by a craniopath who moves cranial bones, then the interlocking bones of the skull will move the bite back out of position, and the dental treatment will need to be redone. The moral of this story is that any work done on the teeth to correct bite imbalances must involve substantial additional therapies to maintain the alignment of the cranial bones. You can find certified craniopaths at the Sacro Occipital Research Society International **www.sorsi.com**

## Jaw Alignment through Body Work

There are several modalities to help your jaw, head and bite all feel more comfortable and function more correctly. Amazingly, each modality which I present here, which I have experienced personally, has a unique perspective on what is important. Each modality generally completely misses something that a practitioner from another modality feels is important. For example, after seeing several experts including an osteopath, several chiropractors from different modalities, and two different cranial sacral therapists, none of them discovered a simple fact that my TMJ joint on the left side was jammed. The next chiropractor I saw, a craniopath, was able to release the locked joint in one or two quick adjustments.[283] While I believe that all these different modalities can learn from one another, and that the specialties could all be involved and enhanced, the reality is most practitioners do not see anything close to the entire picture, and unfortunately many are closed-minded and mired in limiting belief systems even when they offer excellent therapeutic treatments.

The first step to functional orthopedics is nearly always to have body work treatments done. This is my opinion. This is not any official recommendation from any organization. The more treatments, the better. I received body work treatments with a craniopath, a directional non-force chiropractor, and a biodynamic osteopath for about 8 months before getting a dental appliance.[284] I kept receiving the treatments until I would hit a wall in which the treatments were no longer helpful because I needed extra support for my bite from a dental appliance. There are of course other body work modalities and forms of chiropractic work not mentioned here that may help or even completely heal any bite dysfunction.

www.cranialacademy.org—Osteopaths who specialize in the cranial field.

www.nonforce.com—directional non-force chiropractic, especially good with aligning vertebrae.

www.myofascialrelease.com—focuses on releasing tension in the fascia, many Rolfers also work with the fascia.

## Functional Appliances and Practitioners

When I first started searching dentists or functional orthodontists to help correct my bite, I was focused on finding a practitioner who used a specific appliance. This was the wrong way to approach the problem. Dental orthopedics is an art form. You want to search for a functional orthopedist who knows how to use his tools. Having a good saw or a fast drill does not make a good handyman (or a good dentist). Likewise, using a highly reputed technology for bite correction does not necessarily mean the practitioner understands the bite. It is hard to explain this until you actually see it in action. The best of the best functional orthopedists are superlative because they know how to use their tools to produce a result, not because their tools are necessarily advanced or special. Unfortunately, without substantial background education in chiropractic care, physical therapy, craniopathy and osteopathy, dentists are very poorly equipped to correct bite dysfunctions because they never learned how the body functions as a complete organism. They have not been taught how to check for and repair functionality by physically manipulating the patient's body. For example, a chiropractor might muscle test the patient and check for indicators for certain misaligned bones. The chiropractor then adjusts the body accordingly and the bones are realigned. Without having direct hands-on access to the body and without a chiropractor's or osteopath's training in bodywork, the conventional dentist is, in a way, working in the dark. Nothing like this is currently taught in dental school. Conversely, chiropractors and osteopaths are limited in their ability to correct the cranial system and bite of the individual because they have little or no training in orthopedic appliances to overcome physiological obstacles.

The best treatment modalities available therefore are the ones in which the dentist works simultaneously or in close proximity with a cranial expert such as an osteopath. This means literally that an osteopath will be in the office, working with the dentist, helping the dentist fine tune the dental appliance to the patient. This ensures that the dental appliance fits in a way that is beneficial for the patient's body. Without the supplemental bodywork treatments, patients can develop chronic tension and pain as their bodies struggle to adapt to the appliance.

## Functional Dental Appliance Goals

My opinion is that the healthiest and most ideal correction of bite imbalances involves correcting both the height and the width of the bite. The improvement in height and width is in harmony with our therapeutic model of the skulls that show fuller dental arch development. The correct bite height allows the jaw to come forward into the position where the front teeth are completely aligned and with the molars comfortably touching, as demonstrated in figure *a*. The correct bite width widens the maxilla and mandible to allow all of the teeth to fit, including the wisdom teeth. Some critics complain that bite height correction is wrong because it makes the face too long. However if you combine height with width, then the face will look balanced and the head and body will function in a healthier way.

Most of the dental orthopedic work done with children focuses on widening the bite, which is very important but such an approach usually ignores the vertical height aspect. If a child had pretty good vertical height to begin with, as in a minor overbite, then they will have a highly successful outcome from jaw expansion. Children with more severe overbites in which the molar height is more of an issue, will have a less ideal outcome from only expanding the jaw.

## Finding a Functional Orthopedist

You need to be careful as there are some pretty bad functional orthopedists out there, and some appliances that do not work with the natural structure of the body. Even though their treatment paradigm is more correct than conventional orthodontists, you can still suffer from bad treatment outcomes. Too much widening of the jaw, widening the jaw at the wrong rate, or widening at the wrong spot, can all destabilize the cranial system. It is important that the practitioner understands their tools and their art form, and that they are not just using some appliance after a 40-hour training course. Another key to finding a good functional orthopedist is by looking at their treatment outcomes. Do the faces of their patients exhibit aesthetic harmony? Do they look relaxed and natural? Unfortunately there are very few good functional orthopedists, and many times people must travel great distances to see the few good ones available. If your search is long, frustrating, or you do not feel comfortable with the practitioner, you are not alone; it can be a difficult process.

**www.alforthodontics.com**—Advanced Lightwire Functional(ALF) practitioners, some of them work together with osteopaths.

www.aago.com—American Academy of Gnathologic Orthopedics.

www.aacfp.org—American Academy of Cranial Facial Pain.

www.orthotropics.com—Orthotropics, natural growth guidance.

There is also a very interesting new appliance that not many practitioners yet use, called Splint Orthodontic Myofunctional Appliance (SOMA) **www.wholisticdentistry.com.au**

## The End of Braces

Braces are good for rotating teeth which may be twisted and facing the wrong direction, but they are not good tools to widen the jaw. Crooked teeth exist in a mouth that needs more space. When the space is provided through expansion with a functional appliance they will usually straighten on their own. This is working with the body, rather than coercing the teeth to move where the conventional orthodontist thinks the teeth should be. There are some orthodontists who combine dental arch expansion with braces. Some of the case outcomes from some of these practitioners look acceptable. As I said, it is the skill and understanding of the practitioner more than the appliances used that makes the crucial difference. But there are many more elegant solutions than using braces for nearly every type of orthodontic work.

## The Wisdom of Keeping Your Wisdom Teeth

Wisdom teeth are important. They were not put there by accident. As food slides back towards the swallowing position, the back molars chew and crush food. Since wisdom teeth are our third molars, not having wisdom teeth is like losing 25-33% of the chewing surface which you were designed to have. The locations where wisdom teeth were extracted (cavitations) very often become sites for hidden infections.

With dental arch widening, most wisdom teeth can be saved by making space for them with a functional dental appliance. The concept of minimally invasive dentistry is to perform the least amount of surgery, and therefore cause the least amount of trauma, to the jaw and the mouth. Pulling teeth of any kind is not a wise choice, unless there is a severe health-threatening tooth infection, or unrepairable disturbance caused by the wisdom teeth. Just leaving wisdom teeth in there, if there is not enough space for them, may put unnecessary pressure on your trigeminal nerve. When you choose to keep your wisdom teeth, if there is some crowding which is highly common, it would be a good idea to monitor how their roots are growing or expand the jaw to make sure they fit.

There are cases in which removing wisdom teeth seems to be medically required, but usually expanding the jaw is a more prudent approach. It definitely requires more effort and commitment to go through jaw expansion, than just pulling the wisdom teeth out with surgery. Keeping your wisdom teeth will help maintain your ability to chew food, the structure of your face, and your vitality.

# Regaining Your Dental Health

My understanding of bite and how to treat one that is misaligned is a work in progress. Likewise the field of functional orthopedics is an evolving discipline that still has many blind spots and room for growth. The potential for correcting imperfect bites is vast, and the improvements in health and vitality when done properly are well worth it. Our bite is connected to nearly every disease process in the body because of how our nervous system is affected by a poor bite. Like conventional dentistry, conventional orthodontics has failed us miserably. Many times, conventional orthodontics has turned bad dental conditions into worse ones by working against the physiology and natural growth of the body.

Your bite changes how you look. It separates super athletes from mundane individuals because of its effects on the nervous system. Your bite, when it functions properly, can help your teeth remineralize, and it can destroy teeth when it is misaligned. The status of one's bite can be the difference between a vigorous life filled with health and immunity to almost any disease, and a life plagued with discomfort and illness.

*Chapter 10*

# Your Teeth Can Heal Naturally!

## *The Evidence and Proof That Cavities can Remineralize and Heal*

Dr. Price writes regarding the x-rays on the next pages:

> *The pulp chambers and pulp tissues of the root canals are shown as dark streaks in the center of the tooth. The very large cavities that had decalcified the tooth to the pulp chamber are shown as large dark areas in the crown. Temporary fillings had to be placed because of pain produced by the pressure of food on the pulp below the decayed dentine. After the nutrition was improved, the tissues of the pulp built in secondary dentine thus reincasing itself in a closed chamber.*[285]

Dr. Price writes of the ability of teeth to remineralize as a natural result of a diet high in vitamins and minerals:

> *[A] progressive filling in of the pulp chambers can be noted from the deposition of secondary dentine, making a roof over the pulp and thereby providing a protection which enabled the pulp to remain vital and useful for an extended period. This is frequently experienced as a result of reinforcing the diet with high-vitamin and high-activator butter, together with reducing the carbohydrate intake to a normal level as supplied by natural foods and by increasing the foods that provide body-building and tooth-forming miner-als,* **in many cases a hard and even glassy surface resulting.**[286] *(Emphasis added.)*

Dr. Price also shared an example of a 14-year-old girl whose dentist recommended the removal of all of her teeth. After 7 months of a special nutritional program, her teeth were saved and none were removed. (In this case, cosmetic restorations and 4 root canals were still done even though the teeth were saved.)

## Tooth Before (left) and After (right) Nutritional Treatment

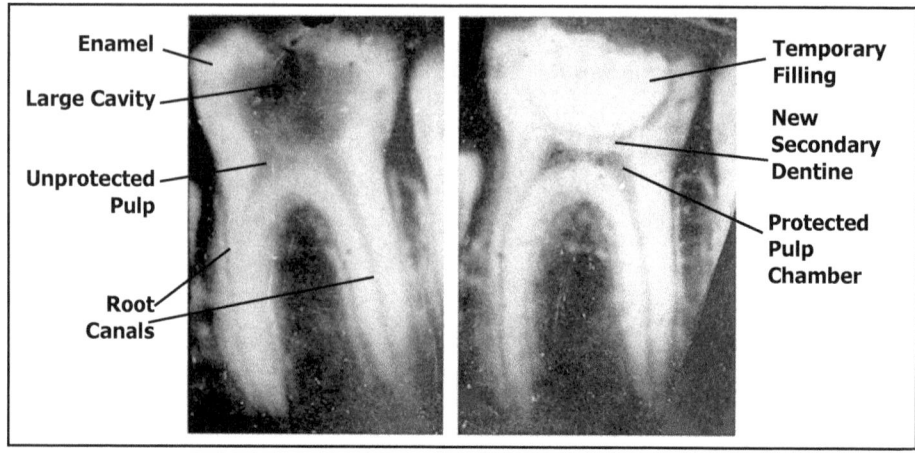

Enamel

Large Cavity

Unprotected Pulp

Root Canals

Temporary Filling

New Secondary Dentine

Protected Pulp Chamber

© *Price-Pottenger Nutrition Foundation, www.ppnf.org*

*When the nutrition is adequately improved, nature can close an exposure of the pulp (due to dental caries) by building a protecting wall within the pulp cham-*

## Child's Permanent Molar Before (left) and After (right) Nutritional Program

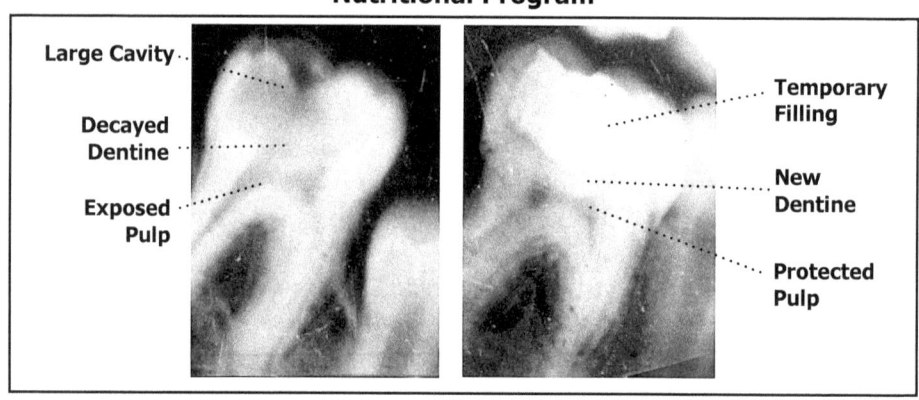

Large Cavity

Decayed Dentine

Exposed Pulp

Temporary Filling

New Dentine

Protected Pulp

© *Price-Pottenger Nutrition Foundation, www.ppnf.org*

*(Left photo) This is a decayed tooth of a child who is at the age where new teeth are coming in. This is prior to a nutritional program. The tooth is a first permanent molar. You can see the dark spot which is the large cavity. The pulp is exposed to the mouth environment, creating pain while chewing. (Right photo) This is the same tooth after a period of nutritional treatment. (Dr. Price did not specify the exact length of time but mentions that the test periods were usually three to five months.) Notice how the new dentin now covers the pulp chamber of the tooth.*

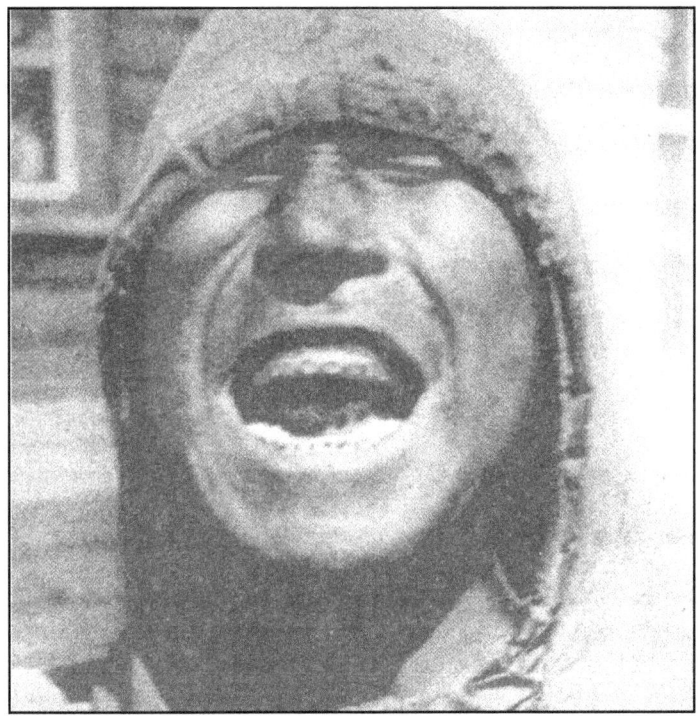

*© Price-Pottenger Nutrition Foundation, www.ppnf.org*
*Typical native Alaskan Eskimo. Note the broad face and broad arches and no dental caries.*[288] *(Original Caption)*

The Inuit people characteristically wore their teeth down as a natural artifact of living their lives, as you can see in the photograph. This wear did not result from tooth decay, but from chewing leather to soften it, and from regularly eating fish and other meat that had collected small bits of sand and grit from being dried in the wind. Due to their excellent diet, the Inuit's teeth constantly repair themselves, such that the pulp chambers and the nerves of the tooth are very well protected. This repair mechanism is not evident in Inuits who abandon their natural diet and switch to one consisting of the foods of modern commerce.

This image serves as further evidence that under excellent nutritional circumstances teeth will rebuild and protect themselves—this is Nature's design.

## Curing Tooth Decay—Parting Words

In several examples throughout this book we have demonstrated that tooth decay is not a result of faulty genetics. Rather, it is primarily the result of the type of food we eat, and the poor management of our body's ecology. Proper health is usually restored to the body through a healing diet, such as a diet based on that of healthy indigenous peoples across the globe. We can reclaim our immunity to tooth decay now and gain other benefits along the way, such as increased overall health, strength, and vitality.

I may have convinced you to begin to take more responsibility for your health and lifestyle habits. And I hope that I have convinced you of the true cause of tooth decay — a deficiency of nutrients, not a lack of fluoride or brushing.

Here are my suggestions for how to begin practicing these habits:

- Align yourself with your intention for health, for the highest good for yourself and for your community. Remind yourself of this several times a day if possible.

- Purchase a good cookbook or two to help you prepare healthy meals. The book _Nourishing Traditions_ by Sally Fallon contains scores of whole-food based recipes, and for those who like raw animal foods I recommend the book Recipe for Living without Disease by Aajonus Vonderplanitz.

- Locate dependable sources for special foods (such as yellow butter, raw milk, liver and bone marrow from grass-fed animals, whole fish including the head and some organs, oysters and so on).

- Eliminate foods on the "avoid list," and begin to replace them with whole-food alternatives as described in the complete tooth decay healing protocol.

# Get Support

To make changes in your diet and improve your health, get additional support. Support can come from a good dentist, a good alternative health practitioner, and/or from friends or family members who regularly eat healthy foods. In particular the Weston A. Price Foundation offers support on finding farm-fresh food, and you can meet people who are cooking in healthier ways. Find your local chapter at: **www.westonaprice.org/localchapters**

## Support with Specific Dental Issues

Please keep in mind that my expertise is in healing and preventing cavities naturally with nutrition. If you have a difficult or painful tooth, I have offered you the best available information on how to heal teeth naturally in this book. My general advice is to take a two-pronged approach to improve your diet as best as you can, and to consult with an excellent dentist on whether specifically damaged teeth need dental treatments, and what type of treatments would be best. Resources in finding an excellent dentist are given in the dentistry chapter. I cannot replace the practical hands-on experience of a good dentist who is required to perform the treatment.

### Book Readers' E-mail List

Readers of this book can sign up on a special e-mail list for book readers only, so I can e-mail you with the latest tips, interviews and important updates to help you stay on top of your cavity healing program.

**www.curetoothdecay.com/subscribe**

## Give Support

Readers like you can make a difference in the world. Portions of this book would not exist if readers had not submitted and shared with me their own knowledge or stories about healing cavities. There are many ways to give back. You can send me your feedback on the book including personal testimonials and expertise, or let me know about unclear parts of the text. You can share this book or the knowledge you have learned with your friends and family. You can show my book to people in the media, or write articles, or share online on social networking sites to help spread the word about healing tooth decay naturally. You can give presentations and teach people how to heal cavities. Regarding any of these pertinent topics, please write to me at: comments@curetoothdecay.com   I will read all of the feedback I receive although it could take four weeks or longer for you to receive a reply depending on if I am traveling.

## Healthy Teeth Are Your Birthright

Let us remember the words of nutrition pioneer Dr. Weston Price:

> *Tooth decay is not only unnecessary, but an indication of our divergence from Nature's fundamental laws of life and health.*[289]

It is true when Dr. Price said that, "Great harm is done, in my judgment, by the sale and use of substitutes for natural foods."[290] There is no other way that I am aware of to be healthy without approaching dental problems directly through improved lifestyle and eating habits. Great harm has been done to our teeth and bones because mere facsimiles of food have replaced real, nutrient-rich food.

In the absence of a dental system that values care, awareness and health, is a conventional dental system of suffering which values secrecy, hiding evidence, false truths, and outwardly hurtful treatments. This tired and destructive way of providing dental care is coming to an end, and thus we find ourselves at a crossroads. This crux relates to a larger story of humanity and our beliefs about ourselves. We are still holding onto the old belief pattern that having a human body is wrong and sinful, and that a better and healthier reality lies somewhere else. Based on this belief system is the justification that humans are meant to suffer because to simply exist, is to be imperfect. If it were true that our purpose is to suffer, then diseases like tooth decay would not be curable. And because of this belief system, its treatments would necessarily involve suffering, pain and disease.

There is a new belief pattern also forming. This belief system affirms that being a human is not wrong or sinful. And therefore if we are suffering, it must not be from our predetermined state of existence, but from self-inflicted suffering from human ignorance. Our suffering is somehow our responsibility. And what is our responsibility lies within our power to change.

We are here to live in Nature's abundance through following Nature's laws. In following these laws we will see that there is no predestined fate of suffering, but rather that human suffering is self-inflicted when we oppose the natural order of life. When we realign with Nature's principles, we connect ourselves with our innate goodness and power to heal, and we move towards balance.

I want to share with you the teachings of our indigenous friends, the Aborigines. Living in harmony with the land and immune to tooth decay, they believed "that life consists in serving others as one would wish to be served."[291] In the absence of the practice of this philosophy, which is also interwoven in many of the world's religions, a system of health care — including dental care — has emerged that is driven more by profit than by the higher motive of service to others. We have all suffered greatly as a result.

I invite you to bring this spirit of service into your life and into the lives of your friends and family. It is this liberator of goodness that has inspired me to create and share with you the possibility of healing your teeth and gums. For I, too, have committed myself to be of service to others, and this book is one of the results.

We can continue to lie and dishonor our own true selves and believe that diseases like tooth decay are not curable. But it is time to move away from this limiting belief. The cause of tooth decay is known: it is a faulty diet. From this knowledge, let us become empowered to take more responsibility for our dental health.

The decision now rests within your hands. Do you take the bold step to ask, "How can I be of service to life?" which of course includes taking excellent care of yourself, your teeth and your gums. Or do you choose the old way of convenience, of using foods that stimulate rather than nourish your body.

Make the commitment to yourself, a commitment to making changes in your diet and lifestyle and let food be your medicine. Yes, it takes work to be healthier and to obtain higher quality foods. But you deserve a healthier life and a healthier mouth. And your community, your friends and family deserve you to be healthy for their sakes as well.

**You are not here to suffer; you are here to heal your suffering!**

Ramiel

# Remineralize and Repair Your Child's Tooth Cavities Naturally

## *Disclaimer for Children's Section*

Your child's health is a delicate matter. This material has been written and published solely for educational purposes and is not intended as a replacement for medical or dental advice. The author and publisher shall have neither liability nor responsibility to any person or entity with respect to any loss, damage or injury caused, or alleged to be caused directly or indirectly by the information contained in this book.

Only you can make the best decisions for your child. I strongly advise you to play an active role and to carefully monitor your child's teeth for decay.

**Note:** The material in this chapter can also be useful for adults healing their own cavities.

## The Depths of Despair

With our daughter facing severe tooth decay, my partner and I both experienced a substantial amount of fear. Watching our daughter's teeth decay before our eyes created a feeling of shock within us. I experienced a tangible terror and sense of powerlessness because my child's body was clearly in less than ideal health. This sinking feeling of fear and helplessness would occur frequently and it is one of the most painful feelings for any parent to experience. Almost every time our daughter pointed to her mouth when she was between 12-20 months old, Michelle and I thought, "Oh no, she has a toothache; what do we do?" If you experience even half of that fear on behalf of your child's health, please know that it is utterly normal to feel this way. Our children are so precious to us; we do not want them to suffer. However, out of the depths of my despair, I have begun to experience my greatest faith and an unsurpassed trust and safety in life, in nature, and in the world.

Many parents are concerned about the long term effects of their children's tooth decay, if the tooth decay is not treated by a dentist with dental surgery. My daughter is now close to seven years old. Her teeth are healthy and pain-free, and her adult teeth are strong, white and cavity-free. I have heard of similar happy outcomes. Many times children with decayed baby teeth will have healthy adult teeth.

# From Fear to Faith, From Suffering to Peace

Here are five strategies that I use to help me find faith, safety, and peace in relation to my daughter's oral health.

## Feel Your Pain

There is something meaningful in feeling the experience you are in, whatever it is. We humans tend to ignore, deny, block, fight against, control, manipulate, and do anything to "fix" the feeling. The feeling that says, "I did something wrong" or "It is my fault" or "Now my child is going to suffer," makes us feel terrible. I want you to allow yourself to feel that feeling. One needs to feel what it is like to be in shock, to be in fear, to be in despair. This is a lesson from life.

Unfortunately, what many parents do is try to eliminate this feeling of fear by doing something that might produce a fast solution. They rush to the nearest dentist to fix their child's teeth. The dentist promises he will help the child; the parent breathes a sigh of relief and believes that they no longer have to feel their inner discomfort and fear. Many adverse circumstances in life are really learning opportunities in disguise. If you ignore your feelings and just attempt to fix the problem, then later other circumstances will trigger the same feelings of pain and a vicious circle will continue until we meet the inner feelings and listen to them. This does not mean you should avoid a dental treatment; I am only encouraging you to look at your feelings first, and then act in a way you believe is healthy. The only way out of the vicious circle is to feel the pain, here and now. Just let go and sink into the feeling. There are no judgments; there is nothing good or bad about your feelings. It is your temporary, momentary truth.

If you get stuck somewhere in these feelings, then you can try prayer or meditation. A simple but effective prayer or meditation might be, "I want to feel all my feelings about this situation." Also, remember to breathe.

If, as a parent, you can tolerate the pain (I am referring to your inner emotional pain) and you do not feel you have to "fix it" in the outer world by immediately engaging all manner of medical procedures, then you have given yourself space to pause and consider. If you are reading this book, then you have given yourself enough inner space beyond the feelings of fear, stress, worry, and so on, to at least explore alternatives to try to choose the best treatment for your child. Try taking a deep breath right now!

Nurturing this inner space is an essential key to making informed and caring choices for your child.

## Intention

What is your intention right now? What is your purpose in reading this book? Are you fully aligned with that intention/purpose? Intention is a place where we have absolute power in our lives. This is where we choose the directions in which we travel. Notice what your current intention is for your children's health; what is it that you want for them? What do you want for yourself? This is important, so take the time to reflect. A sample intention for my daughter is: "I really want her to be healthy." Another intention could be, "I want to treat my child's tooth decay in a way that supports his/her health."

A positive intention is reflected by your willingness to constantly search for the best dental solution relating to your child's health. Pay attention to your intentions.

Many people like to focus on positive intention, but it is also important to notice negative intention, as it can thwart your efforts to stay focused and positive. Negative intention is the intention to be separate and to act out of fearful places within. Some examples of negative intention are laziness or avoidance. It is that inner voice that says, "I do not want to give my best because…I don't have time…it won't work…I cannot do it," and so forth. Each person may have a different voice or inner belief system which can change from time to time. This negative belief resists that natural flow of life towards unity, health and healing. In addition to affirming your positive intention, ferret out those negative places in yourself and acknowledge them so that they will no longer blind you.

## Peer Pressure

Many parents will meet peer pressure concerning the treatment of their children's teeth. For example, someone might ask why you are not brushing or taking care of your child's teeth and thus blame you for your child's tooth decay. I hope you have already come to see that although you were not completely responsible for their condition because society has taught you false beliefs and incorrect prevention methods for tooth decay, you must take complete responsibility for it now. Nobody had educated you on how to prevent tooth decay with good nutrition. You may not have known that brushing is only a secondary factor at best in preventing tooth decay. After reading this book you now understand the essential causes of tooth decay and how to treat them.

It is important to differentiate blame from responsibility. Blame does not have acceptance laced within it. It comes with the connotation that someone is at fault. Parents are often blamed for their child's tooth decay and made to feel as if they are guilty or neglectful. It is important to hold parents accountable and responsible for their child's health, but in an affirming and positive way. You are accountable for what you feed your children and for how you nurture and care for them. Everyone makes mistakes and no one really has the right to blame you.

However, you do need to be accountable for the mistake, educate yourself, and then correct it in the best way possible.

Dentists who treat children may also blame, coerce, emotionally punish, and accuse you as parents. This is done to weaken your resistance to the dentist's demands of an expensive surgical procedure that you are naturally opposed to. If you feel even the slightest bit of this type of stress, confront the dentist and request that he stop. Ask him what evidence he has for these accusations. If he continues this behavior, then please leave and find a better dentist—one who truly wants to help. Remember, you are paying the dentist plenty of money for his expertise and assistance in healing your child's teeth. You are not paying to hear that you are a neglectful parent, nor are you paying him to twist your arm so he can make money with treatments that are not absolutely necessary.

People who tend to blame you will look for anything you are doing that is not in accordance with their beliefs. Usually what they criticize is that you are breastfeeding too much, or not brushing enough. Neither of these allegations can be determined by the dentist or by your peers as truly causing cavities. They cannot determine accurately that you were wrong in your behaviors, and besides, such condemnation only serves destructive ends.

The problem you are facing with peer pressure is a problem of societal ignorance. Many people have rigid beliefs about dentistry and tooth decay that they learned in childhood. Everyone colludes with one another in these belief systems. Thus, rather than expanding their thinking to consider new beliefs that explain how nutritional deficiencies are the primary cause of cavities, people remain mired in the limited belief pattern of blaming bacteria for cavities. In turn, they then blame you for your children's cavities. Blamers hold on to very rigid belief systems, and they are threatened when your behavior puts into question their narrow thinking. Instead, they should be sharing compassion with you about such a challenging and frustrating problem.

Then there is the opposite of peer pressure, which is avoidance of pressure. Many blame "genetics" for their child's decay. Parents can be lazy and claim that decay is inevitable, and that as parents one can do nothing about it. This type of excuse is subtle. It encourages parent not to be responsible for their child's health and it relinquishes one's decision-making power to an authority figure, such as a dentist.

## Cosmetic Appearance

If your child's teeth are decayed, even if they are functional and protected, they may not look very pretty. Your young child, however, thinks everything is beautiful. If her teeth do not conform to the ideal standard of beauty, it won't concern her as long as she is innocent of those standards. Otherwise, the condition of her teeth will seem quite natural and good to her. It is the adult mind and vision that demand a certain cosmetic appearance for our children's teeth. From our conscious and many times limited vision, we may want to hide that our child has tooth decay. I want to encourage you to find beauty in your child's teeth even with the decay. If her teeth have ceased to decay, then they now represent a triumph. They show you what sort of healing is possible, and remind you of how important and cherished your child's health is. When you make the choice about the cosmetics of your child's baby teeth, make the choice that will honor your child and her needs, not one that pays tribute to the adult world filled with superficiality.

## Truth & Knowledge

Within the pages of this book I have provided you with a more accurate view of tooth decay than has been generally presented to the public. This is based upon the physiological and biological processes that occur in the natural world. This information has taken a significant amount of motivation and dedication to find. I have done my best to compile it for you in an easy to understand format so that you can examine it for yourself.

I have demonstrated in my own life that through action and obtaining knowledge we do have power to positively influence our children's health and wellbeing. You can prevent general anesthesia and dental surgery, as well as completely avoid or greatly limit the need for any type of dental treatment on your child's teeth by making wise nutritional choices today. This process may not be the easiest path, but it is definitely possible.

Knowledge can also be used to combat fear. The fear says, "One day my child will have a toothache." But knowledge tells you that today your child is happy and has no toothache. Knowledge and awareness are a part of how I help dissolve the fear. I know that I am giving my child the best foods possible. Her decayed teeth continually remind me of the delicate balance of the foods that are required to keep her healthy.

I remind myself that when I give her these special foods, her body builds defenses against pain, infection, and decay. If I experience fear, when in the real world there is nothing to fear, then I have to challenge and examine that fear. If it arises when my daughter is not experiencing pain or discomfort, I choose to seek out its origins within me. Where did it come from? How do I justify it? What am I afraid of, and how can I hold a compassionate and aware presence in the face of this fear?

Knowledge is also obtained by examining your child's tooth decay and closely monitoring it. Most people are better off monitoring tooth decay with a dentist, but I understand the difficulty this poses in some cases and people have had problems finding supportive dentists that are open to the "watch and wait" approach. "Watch and wait" used to be the way children's cavities were treated. If the tooth got infected, the tooth was simply pulled out, and although that is not a pleasant procedure, it is short and quick. There was no drama about general anesthesia surgery, no metals placed in the child's mouth, and plenty of patience in monitoring a little decay in a baby tooth.

# Children's Tooth Decay is Not an Easy Road for Most

For many parents, including myself, dealing with children's tooth decay is not an easy thing. It can challenge you at the deepest level. Today, I still find myself occasionally overly concerned about my daughter's teeth. I still feel that twinge of fear within me that says, "Her teeth are not sound enough as they are." One day my daughter complained of a minor toothache. Because I was carefully monitoring her diet, I knew the cause and I knew how to stop it. She had been eating too much raw honey. The honey had caused her blood sugar to be elevated for too long, and thus her blood levels of calcium and phosphorus became imbalanced, resulting in decay. We began to be more careful and restrictive about the honey and other sweets in her diet. That was over a year ago and she has not had a toothache since. Removing the honey caused her blood chemistry to remain balanced, and thus her tooth remineralized and the pain stopped.

Several years ago, my daughter apparently had a tooth infection and was restless for several nights. One day she woke up with a slightly swollen face. I thought to myself, "This is not good." In the midst of my nervousness and discomfort at the sight of my daughter's partially swollen face, Michelle added her words of wisdom and said, "Don't worry about it." I exclaimed, "What do you mean 'Don't worry'?!" I expressed my fear that this was the worst thing that we had come up against. Upon review of the past several days, we together saw that our hurried ways, our laziness, and our hunger had resulted in improper food preparation. This chain of events leading up to the infection was clearly the cause. We had allowed our daughter to eat too many grain products of mediocre quality. The day we saw the infection we immediately put her on a food protocol similar to the best protocol which I describe in this book. The diet included fish (cooked and raw), oysters, eggs, some bacon, vegetables, vegetable juice, cod liver oil and butter oil. We greatly limited sweet foods, were careful about grain products, and we made sure to establish boundaries so that she had balanced meals. Gradually over a few days, the swelling disappeared and the abscess healed. Not all parents need to work this hard to prevent their child's tooth decay. It really depends on how fragile their child's body and system are.

I continue to learn lessons from these experiences. I am learning that we need to be vigilant concerning our family's diet. I continue to challenge myself to feel the fear, to experience that "what if" scenario that my mind always worries about. Then I also begin to experience periods of feeling great happiness and satisfaction. There are times when I can move beyond the emotional fear and see my daughter's tooth decay in an honest and mature way. I trust and understand this part of life because I have faced it emotionally, through feeling my feelings, mentally, through knowledge and research; and I have faced it with my will, through taking positive steps to treat her condition. That is how I have found safety and peace in the face of illness. The result is a happy and carefree child, free from tooth pain.

# Treating Children's Tooth Decay Naturally

We have successfully treated severe early childhood tooth decay for five years now, without fluoride, dentists, or dental surgery. I estimate we have achieved about a 90-98% reduction in the rate of tooth decay. Many parents have achieved 100% or more reduction in tooth decay, by which I mean the complete cessation of cavities, and even occasionally the disappearance of previously visible tooth decay. How successful you will be is a factor of how committed you are to health, the quality of foods that are available, your ability to maintain a healthy diet for your child, and how severely deficient your child was when you begin the program of improvement.

One of my daughter's baby teeth is black and worn to the gum line. Even with this, her gums are healthy, with no sign of infection, or pain. Her adult teeth do not have any cavities.

# Surgery on Children for Tooth Decay?

In the U.S., 27.9% of all children ages 2–5 have had some tooth decay, with a total average of about 5 out of every 100 teeth in young children exhibiting signs of some tooth decay.[292] Young children cannot sit still in order to undergo normal dental procedures. Until the child is somewhere around the age of 6–8 years, the child is not really capable of understanding what a dental procedure is.

A mother's lap can be appropriate for certain dental treatments which are done quickly, but not for substantial dental treatments. Many mothers will find that their toddler will protest sitting in a dental chair. Some may not even open their mouths. Young children are fearful of the dentist putting his hands or cold, hard metal instruments into their mouths. Young children do not have the cognitive ability to fully comprehend what is happening. Their interpretation of the experience is that some strange person is shining bright lights at them and forcing them to do things which are uncomfortable and invasive. This makes it challenging to treat young children's teeth without violating their will and without causing them pain or fear. Forcing the child to go through dental procedures before he is ready may cause emotional trauma.

Local anesthesia may not work on young children. It may or may not be effective in preventing pain and it is difficult to tell if a young child's tooth is numbed properly prior to dental surgery. This is because it is almost impossible to get reliable feedback from a child if they are under stress, especially if they are younger than six.

Treating children as if they are mini adults is a backwards way to go about dentistry, but this is the common pediatric dentistry model. This means that dentists will use crowns, root canals, and fillings in a vain attempt to try to remove the infestation of bacteria on a child's teeth. If the child's cavities are extensive, dentists recommend significant surgery for decayed baby teeth. The two common methods of pediatric dentistry for children with significant tooth decay are barbaric. One is to heavily sedate the child with an oral sedative. The child is still awake, just immobile and groggy. It is common for many dental offices then to strap the drugged child to the dental chair in order to restrain the child during treatment, including drilling. The other method is administration of full general anesthesia, in which the child is separated from the parents, put to sleep while teeth are extracted and typically metal is placed into the child's mouth. Some children may be able to cope with these harrowing experiences, but for many others they may cause indelible emotional scars.

I told a friend from another country that this is how they treat children with several tooth cavities in dental offices in the U.S. She thought I was joking at first because she could not believe parents would submit their children to such a procedure, nor that dentists would even offer it. I understand surgery with general anesthesia if a child has a life-threatening medical condition, but for tooth decay? No way.

Since young children's bodies are immature and delicate, the administration of general anesthesia comes with the risk of death. This risk of death seems to be quite low for young children although it does happen. I could not find a reliable and conclusive statistic on what the percentage is. With adults the risk of death during dental surgery using anesthetics is extremely small.[293] There is an approximate 35% risk of an adverse event (other than death) from general anesthesia on young children, which is about twice the risk for adults.[294] Furthermore, recent experiments on lab rats have shown that anesthesia, when used while the brain is developing, causes neurodegeneration;[295] that is, a degradation of the nerves that can lead to subtle but prolonged changes in behavior, including memory and learning impairments. I did read one case study of a child who died after dental surgery with general anesthesia, probably because his body had an allergic reaction to the numerous metal crowns placed in his mouth.

The horrors of neurodegeneration are above and beyond the emotional shock and pain of the disassociated feelings caused by the anesthetic. Furthermore, as a result of being so young and vulnerable, along with the added intoxication from the drugs, children will not understand what is happening to them. As the young child is being put under anesthesia, they may experience traumatic separation

## Surgery vs. Nutritional Healing

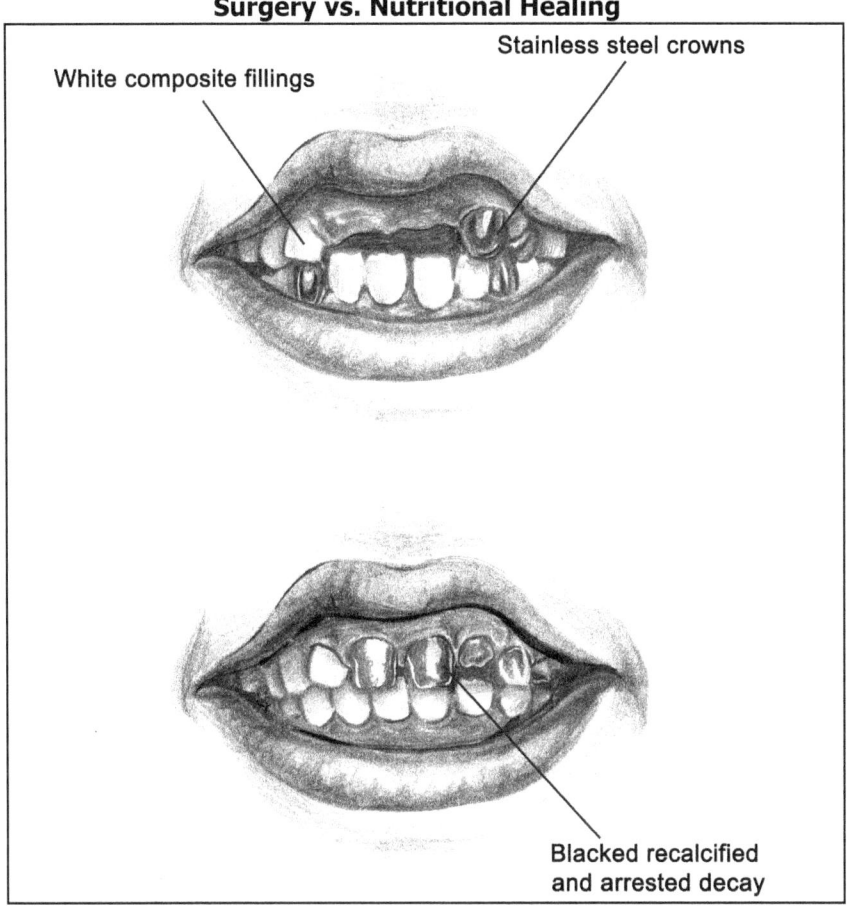

White composite fillings

Stainless steel crowns

Blacked recalcified
and arrested decay

Above: *A typical young child's mouth after dental surgery for severe decay. The front four teeth have been pulled, composite fillings have been placed where decay is less severe, and steel crowns where decay is more severe.*

Below: *When tooth decay is arrested the secondary dentin hardens and can turn black. This option is more humane than surgery*

from their parents. Other emotional traumas may occur during this time when they are helpless and drugged.

As with the rest of conventional dentistry, the profit motive is a significant factor in diagnosing and performing surgery with general anesthesia on children. With a fee of $2,000–$6,000 US dollars per surgery, pediatric dental surgery is a lucrative business. As a result I recommend people look for dentists for their children who do not perform full anesthesia surgery.

*Surgery with General Anesthesia is not an Effective Treatment*

After dental surgery with general anesthesia:

> 23% of all children require further extractions and restorations.
>
> 52% of children have a relapse within 4-6 months.
>
> 57% have new cavities in 6-24 months (different study).[296]

The statistics show us that surgery under general anesthesia is largely ineffective in curing tooth decay. This is because it does not address the real cause, the nutrient imbalance in the child's diet.

## Toxic Dentistry in Children's Mouths

Stainless steel jackets placed in children's mouths contain nickel. Nickel creates a negative electrical current in the mouth[297] and is highly toxic to the nervous system. Nickel may be related to arthritis, and some types of cancer such as lung and breast. [298] In fact, nickel is used to induce cancer in laboratory animals.[299]

Everything you learned from the dentistry chapter applies doubly to children. Children's developing immune and detoxification systems have fewer defenses against toxic assaults. Most dental procedures are toxic to children because of the materials used. Conversely there is no evidence of the safety of these materials for use in children. Just because a dentist uses certain materials regularly does not mean that they have been proven to be safe.

There are also other dental treatments on children that you should not allow. Any type of metal restorations, such as stainless steel crowns or mercury-laden amalgams, has a chance of causing significant problems to your child's health. An example of one such case involved a child whom doctors believed was ill with leukemia but in reality was suffering from heavy metal poisoning due to the nickel in her stainless steel crowns.[300] Do not ever put an amalgam or stainless steel in your child's mouth.

## England's Dentists say, "No Benefits, no Proof, and no Evidence" to support ANY dental Treatment on Painless Baby Teeth

The overarching goal for any type of treatment, surgical or nutritional, for your child's cavities is to keep your child healthy and pain free. But there is no scientific evidence that any drilling, filling, crown, or root canals performed on a painless baby tooth has any impact on the longevity of the tooth, or whether the child experiences future pain. Yes, you heard me correctly; as a preventative measure there is no documented evidence to show any benefits for any dental treatments on baby teeth for tooth decay.[301] This finding is only logical since I have shown you how tooth decay is not cured by dentistry, and that many times dentistry itself renders our teeth in worse shape by the loss of healthy tooth tissue to the aggressive dental drill.

A meeting of over 50 practicing dentists at the University of Manchester in England in 2009 found that treating baby teeth with cavities that do not cause pain achieved nothing other than exposing the child to the drill, and to discomfort.[302] Further, there was no difference between the amount of pain or extractions in teeth with or without dental treatments.[303] This certainly proves that performing dental treatments on children to prevent tooth pain or infection is an exercise in futility. Such an approach is not in concert with the intention of keeping your child's teeth healthy or pain free. This is because the real cause of cavities is never addressed, and the dental treatment simply hides the problem without providing protection against cavities.

In a study of 481 children, ages 1–12, it was found that after taking certain factors into consideration, 82% of decayed baby teeth fell out without pain. 18% of children experienced pain in their untreated teeth. The teeth most likely to cause pain were molars of children showing decay before the age of three years.[304] Children who were older and developed cavities in their baby teeth were less likely to experience pain from the carious teeth.

In a 2003 study of children's tooth decay, published in the *British Dental Journal*, the authors write:

> *More disturbing perhaps, was the discovery that increased levels of restorative care in children were not associated with fewer episodes of pain or the need for extraction.*[305]

The authors of this article bring up the essential question:

> *Do we actually know the best way to care for children with decay in the primary dentition?*[306]

The purpose of this article was to point out that, in relation to tooth decay, we do not utilize the best methods for the care of our children. As a result of our cultural ignorance, laziness, and hidden cruelty, our children have suffered needlessly. The authors continue, regarding children's restorations:

> *We have no scientifically rigorous comparative data on the prevalence of pain and discomfort and longer term outcome measures associated with teeth restored with stainless steel crowns and amalgam.*[307]

To put it plainly, we have not performed the scientific case studies to prove dental procedures actually reduce or prevent pain in our children's baby teeth. A tooth treated with dental fillings may continue to cause a child mild discomfort or cause even more discomfort than an untreated decayed tooth.

# Healing Early Childhood Tooth Decay Naturally

The reason dental surgery does not usually cure dental problems is because modern dental treatments treat the symptoms of the problem (rotting teeth) but do not treat the root of the problem (diet). Many dentists offer the preventative treatment of fluoride, but fluoride is a deadly poison and when fluoride is being placed in our water, our toothpastes, and on our teeth it adds a toxic burden to the body. Because of their less developed immune systems, children are more susceptible to chemical exposure than adults. It is risky and unwise to expose your child to fluoride at a young age.

## Dental Treatments for Infants', Toddlers' and Young Children's Teeth

Using the dental scientific research from England which has found that dental treatments offer no preventative help for tooth pain or infections we can develop a good outline on how to deal with cavities in young children's teeth. These suggestions are not meant to replace your own personal desires for your child's teeth; they are meant to help you find how you really want to take care of your child's teeth. For a child who is too young to sit comfortably still to receive a dental treatment, the treatment paradigm is simple. Consider the very protocol that old school dentists, those who have been in practice 30 years or longer, have learned to rely upon. Keep a close eye on the decayed baby teeth with your dentist. If there is an infection, or tooth pain that does not clear up, then consider pulling the tooth as a last resort treatment. If the tooth is causing pain and can be repaired with a filling rather than an extraction then a biocompatible filling might be useful in that circumstance if the child will cooperate with the treatment. Otherwise, consider leaving the teeth as they are, and use nutrition to prevent tooth pain, cavities, and infections. If you leave decayed teeth as they are, they will need to be closely monitored.

## Dental Treatments on Older Children's Teeth

With older children who can sit still in a dental chair, you have more treatment options to consider. Once they are past the age of five or six, the odds of them experiencing tooth pain from tooth decay is decreased. In this age group, there are some teeth, especially those causing pain, which will benefit from a biocompatible filling to stop tooth pain. Again your treatment choices are your decision; you must weigh your specific needs and circumstances and use your own best judgment on how to proceed.

# Why Do Children Have Cavities?

Several months before the conception of your child, the stage for his or her health was set. The diet and overall health of both the father and the mother-to-be, before conception, was a primary determinant for the physical health of your child. With our modern deficient diet, the mother's body and the father's seed often lack the resources of vitamins and nutrients to create a strong and robust child. After the child is born, during his or her first few years of life, he or she goes through very rapid stages of growth. This growth occurs in spurts and during these growth spurts there is an additional need for vitamins and minerals. The body stores nutrients for these growth spurts, and then grows quickly as it uses nutrient stores. During these rapid growth spurts, if nutrients are missing in body, the needed minerals and building blocks are pulled from the teeth. Another cause of tooth decay is when children are fed too many sweet foods and their body chemistry falls out of balance, resulting in tooth destruction.

## Weak Teeth from Birth

Dr. Mellanby's experiments on canine teeth reveal the effect of a pregnancy diet on children's teeth.. Weak, or hypoplastic, teeth in young children is a common problem which is related to the diet of the mother during pregnancy. Female dogs that were fed a good diet during pregnancy had puppies that even when given a poor diet, were highly immune to cavities because they had been born with well-built teeth. When female dogs were fed a poor diet during pregnancy, and their puppies were given a poor diet, the puppies usually formed cavities because the teeth were weak since birth.[308] This demonstrates that the conditions before and during pregnancy can substantially affect how susceptible your child is to tooth decay now. The good news is that even weak teeth can be made strong, but the diet of a child with weak teeth will need to be more closely monitored than that of a child born with strong teeth.

# Dietary Keys for Remineralizing Tooth Decay in Young Children

Healing children's cavities is essentially the same as healing adult cavities.

- Add fat-soluble vitamins into the diet, particularly vitamins A, D and Activator X.

- Increase dietary minerals particularly calcium and phosphorous.

- Balance blood sugar with low sugar meals and adequate levels of protein throughout the day.

- Avoid toxic and denatured foods; avoid whole grain foods with bran.

One nutritional requirement for infant health is iron. Many times mothers who are vegan, vegetarian, or eat little meat, are the mothers of children who have severe childhood tooth decay. In considering the cause of my daughter's tooth decay, I point to the mostly vegetarian diet followed by Michelle and myself, before and during pregnancy. Thankfully, we occasionally ate fish. Breast milk does not have any viable amount of iron and after six months of age the infant has exhausted her body's iron stores. Not by coincidence, this is the age when infants can eat their first foods. Most likely, feeding infants and toddlers mashed vegetables and fruit does not provide adequate absorbable iron. As a result, their blood does not remain strong and they lose their ability to grow healthy teeth.

Feeding young children pre-chewed or blended grass-fed liver, grass-fed lamb, grass-fed beef, or fresh clams from clean waters will help provide them with adequate amounts of utilizable iron. How you prepare the food for your child is your choice. A majority of people will want to offer their children cooked vegetables and cooked proteins. This is fine, especially in the form of soups and stews with bone broth. Just as with adults you will want to avoid feeding your child too many raw, cellulose-rich vegetables. You can do this by cooking vegetables or juicing them (provided you understand which vegetables are low in antinutrients when raw like celery, cucumber, parsley and cilantro). A few parents like to go the raw or rare route for dairy and animal proteins; this is also fine. Use your best judgment and the feeding principles that you feel comfortable with. As long as your child can digest the food properly, it will add to his health.

# A Food guide for Halting Childhood Tooth Decay

Young children can be finicky eaters. I follow the principle of never forcing children to eat anything. However sometimes they need strong encouragement to eat certain foods we know are good for them to help shift their metabolism and body chemistry in a new direction. Encouraging children to drink milk for strong bones and good health used to be a habit in the United States when the milk was farm fresh and usually raw. That habit died as the quality of milk deteriorated.

## *Fat-Soluble Vitamins Every Day*

You will want to ensure that your child receives the important fat-soluble vitamins for teeth every day as discussed in chapter three on fat-soluble vitamins. I recommend the Blue Ice™ Royal Blend because it is so easy to give the fat-soluble vitamins they need. The amount of Blue Ice™ Royal Blend from Green Pasture (can be purchased at **codliveroilshop.com**) you give to your child depends on the health, nutrient deficiency, and weight of your child. You will need to use your best judgment based upon the dosage of a teenager. For severe cavities a teenager or adult dosage is $\frac{1}{2}$ of a teaspoon of a mixture of cod liver oil and butter oil 2–3 times per day to comprise a total of 1 to $1\frac{1}{2}$ teaspoons per day.

You will need to adjust these daily doses based on your intuition or with the guidance of a health practitioner. These are based upon weight of your child.

Estimated daily dosages of the butter and fermented cod liver oil mixture:

25 pounds:  $\frac{1}{4}$ teaspoon per day

35 pounds:  $\frac{1}{3}$ teaspoon per day

45 pounds:  $\frac{1}{2}$ teaspoon per day

55 pounds:  $\frac{2}{3}$ teaspoon per day

If you want or need to use other sources of fat-soluble vitamins then you will want to give your child as much as they like to eat of vitamin A-rich foods like liver, vitamin D-rich foods like egg yolks and lots of oily fish, and Activator X-rich foods like yellow butter. Bone marrow and fish eggs also are excellent sources of fat-soluble vitamins for healing children's cavities. For added fat-soluble nutrient support my family uses fermented skate liver oil. Skate liver oil offers some unique vitamins that seem to strengthen the overall health of many children.

## Excellent Foods

Feed these foods to your children in proportion to their appetite for them. You can also take advice from the tooth decay healing food suggestions in chapter five. Below is a summary of some foods that can be especially helpful to have in your diet.

Bone broths or homemade soups and gravies made with them are excellent for children.

Raw grass-fed whole fat milk, butter, cream and cheese. Cheese is particularly dense in calcium and phosphorous.

Soft-boiled pastured eggs or yolks, or raw eggs in a smoothie.

Cooked or raw fish is especially potent in reducing tooth decay. Include oysters and clams.

Delicately cooked grass-fed beef and/or lamb.

Tallow, duck fat, or lard from grass-fed animals.

Wild-caught fish eggs.

## *Balancing Foods*

Feed your child fermented foods such as fermented sweet potatoes, sauerkraut, yogurt and kefir to help balance digestion.

Cooked vegetables, such as zucchini, string beans, kale, and chard. Add plenty of butter and/or cream.

Seaweeds of every sort; they are high in macro and trace minerals.

Vegetable juice if you know which vegetables do not contain anti-nutrients or the Ayurvedic green cooked vegetable soup or smoothie.

## *Foods to Avoid*

Avoid all packaged food and processed baby and children's food. Make all of your baby food at home.

Do not serve any processed foods on the "avoid list" in chapter 6.

Avoid infant formula. Use raw milk or bone broth formula instead.

Whole grains, oatmeal, breakfast cereals and granola.

Refined sweeteners containing fructose.

**Vaccines and pharmaceuticals.**

## *Foods to Limit and Be Aware Of*

How strict you need to be with your child's diet really has to do with how severe their cavities are. For children with active and severe decay, limit sweet foods to one meal per day or omit altogether. Make sure the sweet food is natural…like fruit. When they are healthy, more fruits are acceptable, but you must pay close attention to how fruit consumption affects their health. Do not give your child sweetened foods and fruits throughout the day, as this will cause excess blood sugar fluctuations. You will notice that many store-bought baby foods are made with fruits that are very sweet.

**Natural sweets that can promote tooth decay.** Any natural sweetener such as cane sugar, stevia, maple syrup, unheated honey, bananas, sweet apples, oranges, grapes, peaches, pineapples, cherries, dates, raisins, dried fruit, and other very sweet fruits that are not listed here.

**Potatoes.** Potatoes that are not fermented may contribute to tooth decay.

**Beans.** It is unclear whether beans in the diet of young children supports their health.

**Safer sweet fruits.** Cooked fruit seems to be better than raw fruit in terms of sugar content. We use fruits like berries, pears, kiwis, and apples sparingly. If you have been feeding your child sweet foods frequently, such as maple syrup at breakfast, honey at lunch, and fruit and ice-cream at dinner, then your child might have a detoxification response to having the sugar removed. As with quitting a powerful drug, he will have to experience some discomfort and may protest as his body adjusts to a healthier diet.

**Vegetables.** While vegetables are a balancing food, never force your child to eat vegetables. Cooked and raw vegetables may have nutrients that are difficult for some children to utilize.

## Whole Grains and Childhood Tooth Decay

In reviewing my older daughter's own case of severe cavities, I found several photos of her consuming whole grain products we made at home. The grain foods were usually from freshly ground organic grains which were soaked overnight prior to cooking. The whole grains were even consumed in the context of a nutrient-rich diet high in fat-soluble vitamins.

Toxins in grains, whether it is phytic acid, lectins or other compounds, can cause severe cavities quite rapidly. A severe case of cavities in a five-and-a-half-year-old girl was related to me from a Canadian correspondent which illustrates the point. The mother took the child to her dentist regularly every 6 months for the child's entire life. She submitted the child to dental surgery under general anesthesia and spent thousands of dollars on her dental treatments. Yet even after all of this, the child needed four more root canals, three more crowns and five new fillings. A severe case like this is not the result of a high sugar diet, but the result of a potent toxin in grains. When questioned about the girl's diet, the mother told me that the girl received, along with nut butters, seeds, and sweet fruits, a daily supplement of wheat bran and wheat germ in her morning smoothies.

I have studied the diets of several cases of children and adults with rampant cavities. Severe cavities behave like an unending torrent of decay which seems impossible to stem as new cavities rapidly form. One tooth may have multiple cavities, and nearly every tooth is infected with tooth decay. Under most circumstances, it is quite difficult to cause this sort of rampant severe tooth decay in such a brief period of time. For example, in adults, drinking multiple cans of decay-causing soft drinks every day over a period of several years will produce severe cavities. A diet consisting of a large percentage of fruit over a period of many years in one case produced ten cavities. Yet in a relatively short period of time, whole grains can cause severe cavities in children with hypoplastic (weak) teeth from birth.

Young children cannot digest modern grains well. A good suggestion is to wait until they are one or two years old to feed them any grains at all. Always avoid white flour, crackers and store-bought breakfast cereals. Avoid any grains containing bran. The exception may be pseudo-cereals like buckwheat and quinoa. If your child has significant cavities I would not recommend feeding any grains to your child until the severe tooth decay has stopped. If a child has minor tooth decay, then you can feed the safe grains as discussed in chapter four, such as sourdough bread from unbleached flour, or correctly prepared rice. Sprouted grain breads are not helpful for any child with cavities because of their bran content.

## Severe Tooth Decay and Children

Children with a weak constitution or ones who develop cavities easily many times have been exposed to toxins from the bran and germ in grains, or to an extremely inferior diet such as a vegan diet filled with lots of sweet foods. Because these children face a large nutritional deficiency, you will need to be extremely vigilant to heal these types of cavities. If whole grain consumption (no matter how you prepared it) is the cause, then your child will be hypersensitive to most grains. I recommend at least avoiding all grains for 3 weeks for a child with pain or severe tooth decay. You will want to focus on increasing calcium in the diet such as from cheese, and vitamin D such as from fermented cod liver oil, and vitamin C from vegetable or berry sources. These children will do better on a lower grain and lower carbohydrate diet. Their diet will therefore focus primarily on vegetables, with animal proteins and fats. You can use sweet potatoes, other root vegetables, or dairy products to provide them with carbohydrates.

## Tooth Infections and Tooth Pain

A young child with severe decay can develop infections in the gum as a result of compromised teeth. The infections come and go and are usually a result of poor food choices by the parents. The white pus is a sign that the rest of the body will be protected. With improved diet, tooth infections normally heal. **Echinacea with goldenseal tincture diluted in water can help heal tooth and gum infections**. This is to be taken internally by both the child and breastfeeding mother. I have seen echinacea perform wondrous healing of infections. Goldenseal powder or plantain powder can be placed on the infected gum itself. Again use herbs with care. Try a very small dose at first to make sure your child doesn't react adversely to it, and make sure not to use these herbs with prescription medications or other strong herbs unless advised to do so by a practitioner.

You can learn more about tooth infections in the dentistry section. The same general principles apply to children. Make sure to closely monitor teeth that can become infected. Infected teeth that do not heal properly can result in bone loss, or the child getting sick from a focal infection. Infected teeth that do not heal or improve in a short period of time usually need to be extracted. If the pain and infection do not go away and stay away then this is a sign that the body is not able to heal the damaged tooth. Remember there could be years of deficiency that have caused the tooth to break down. While I would not recommend pulling teeth as a preventative measure since there is no evidence to support this, pulling out painful teeth or ones where the infection does not heal quickly can be a good idea. This is your decision to make along with your dentist. You know what is right to do, so trust your own feelings on the matter.

## Moderate Tooth Decay in Children

Not all children require heroic measures to restore their dental health. It really depends on how strong they are, and how many cavities they have. Children with a few small cavities will respond very well to a moderate amount of dietary modifications. In particular, adding fat-soluble vitamins into the diet, and getting good quality raw milk or cheese is usually sufficient to remineralize small cavities in children's teeth. This along with avoiding too many sweets is a good place to begin if you feel unable or unwilling to completely clean up your child's diet.

## Junk Foods in Schools, at Parties and Gatherings

There are two types of sweet foods. There are sweets that in moderation do not harm healthy children who have no tooth decay, and then there are just plain harmful sweets. Occasionally having sweet fruit or natural sugar in a dessert does not harm a healthy child. But many children are exposed to high intensity sweeteners with high fructose corn syrup (corn sugar). When children eat these foods at parties, such as ice cream, or cake, it throws their body chemistry into a tail spin. Children with tooth decay can be adversely affected by these sweets for weeks and months. When well-meaning adults at schools, community gatherings or birthday parties feed children high intensity sweeteners, they are poisoning them with highly toxic artificial food. This is not acceptable behavior from organizations that are supposed to support and safeguard children's health and safety. Be vigilant about keeping these sweets away from your child especially if he has tooth decay.

## Grains You Can Feed Your Children

If your child's cavities have remineralized and you believe the original cavities were not caused by too many whole grains, then you can safely feed your child grains as discussed in the previous chapters. Likewise if your child has a strong and robust constitution and the tooth decay is not too bad, you can follow the grain guidelines for adults. If your child has more severe cavities or other damage from grains, you will need to be very careful with any grains you feed your child for many years, and in this case, grains should be used minimally.

## Vegetarian Children

Vegetarian children should follow a diet similar to the diet in the vegetarian section. I would encourage a parent whose child is vegetarian and has severe cavities to consider some sea food or cod liver oil. Green Pasture's™ butter oil is a must for vegetarian children because they will otherwise be lacking in fat-soluble vitamin D.

## Dairy-Free Diets for Children

Since children with tooth decay may be lacking calcium, having dairy foods in the diet is extremely helpful in healing tooth cavities. If your child is sensitive to dairy foods, see if kefir, goat milk, or some type of grass-fed cheese is comfortable for them to eat. If your child absolutely cannot tolerate dairy products, then you will need to get calcium from sea foods and vegetables. In this case you will need to prepare vegetable soups and stews, preferably with a meat or fish stock base to provide adequate calcium. The calcium guidelines in chapter four will help you with more suggestions for calcium-rich foods.

## Feeding Children Who Won't Eat Good Food

Children mirror and mimic their parents' food habits. Pay attention to the foods you eat and you might find that even though you may eat meat or eggs, you could be a finicky eater and consume too many foods that are not in balance with your needs. While these habits may not affect you overtly, they affect your child to a greater degree. Sometimes children won't eat meat if they have a chronic feeling of pain and emotional upset. If a parent smiles and enjoys a particular food, then the child will usually follow. Sometimes you will need to be positively assertive to persuade your child to eat certain foods. A small struggle may ensue while you help your child switch from addictive, less healthy foods, and you may need many days to completely make the change. Children who do not digest foods high in phytic acid such as grains, beans, nuts, and seeds often have an aversion to eating proteins and fats. You will have to eliminate the foods that are not being digested well in order for them to eat meat. Herbs or homeopathy can also be used to help rebalance a child's constitution.

# Vaccines Promote Tooth Decay

There is evidence in studies performed on dogs that implicates vaccines in the formation of tooth decay. I know of one case of significant tooth decay in a young girl that was traced to a DPT vaccine. Vaccines contain many neurological poisons. Vaccine ingredients include ethylene glycol (antifreeze), formaldehyde, aluminum, thimerosal (mercury), neomycin (anti-biotic), streptomycin(anti-bacterial), squalene (fish, or plant oil), gelatin, MSG, phenol(a caustic, poisonous acidic compound present in coal tar and wood tar).

When the body faces an onslaught of injected carcinogens, vital organs can lose some of their functional ability. The modified proteins and DNA strands may bind to or clog the villi in the intestine, restricting food absorption. Vaccination makes children weaker and more prone to tooth decay because vaccines mostly consist of poisons and toxic material. While this is not a full discussion of vaccinations, there are no reputable double blind studies to show that they work or that they are safe. In other words there is no evidence of their success. Vaccines can promote tooth decay by unbalancing the body chemistry as the body tries to cope with this toxic burden. Seek natural replacements and alternatives.

Learn more about vaccines at:

**www.healingourchildren.net/vaccine_side_effects.htm**

Other drugs may also cause or promote tooth decay including antibiotics.

## How to Prevent Cavities in Babies

What conventional dentists do not know is that the key to preventing cavities in children is not found in genetics, but in the parents' diet prior to conception. Prior to conception, the mother and father need to avoid the industrialized foods that make us sick and depleted. At the same time, they need to regularly consume plenty of fat-soluble vitamins and avoid the bran and germ of most grains. During pregnancy the mother needs to have the same fat-soluble-rich food and limit her exposure to grain anti-nutrients and sweets.

During breastfeeding and the early years of the child, a diet of nutrient-rich whole foods that contain fat-soluble vitamins should continue.

I have created a free website that presents in more detail some factors to consider for preconception health. **www.preconceptionhealth.org**

## What You Can Expect from Nutritional Treatments

Treating tooth decay with nutrition means that children will not suffer from pain or dental infections. The teeth will become hard and resilient, as they are meant to be. In some cases of severe cavities the rapid and severe tooth decay can be slowed down, but not totally stopped in the short term. Even when the decay is not entirely halted and seems to slightly progress, new tooth dentin can still form and your child's teeth can be protected from breaking and from infection of the tooth root.

The teeth rarely if ever fill in; they can only remineralize over the surface of the decayed area. The tooth may have a hole, but the tooth root and pulp will be protected by the hard dentin, the middle tooth layer. My daughter has two primary teeth worn to the gum line. They are little more than black spots. The black color and hard texture indicates arrested tooth decay. Her teeth are hard to the touch, even the black ones.

## Monitoring Your Child's Tooth Decay

The best way to monitor tooth decay in a child is with the help of a good dentist. If you look at an x-ray or diagram of a tooth, you will see that at least 50% of the tooth structure is below the gum line. That means that even badly decayed teeth may have significant and even healthy tooth structure below the gum line. The health of the gums around the decayed tooth is one indication of whether or not the tooth is healthy below the gum line. Pink, firm gums are healthy; bleeding or inflamed gums would indicate less health.

To monitor healing of tooth decay at home, use an explorer, a tool with a pointed end that is not sharp, but strong enough so that you can probe the decayed area and see if it is soft, or hard and glassy.

You also can learn whether or not dietary intervention is working if your child seems happier and is vibrant with plenty of energy. Whining, constant complaining and lethargy are all signs your child is still deficient in nutrients. Take digital pictures of your child's teeth so that you have a visual chart for reference.

### Children's Dentists

Many parents have a difficult time finding a dentist they can trust for their children. Parents are better off working with a good dentist. However I understand that you may not find one who works well with your child and desires. I suggest that you take care of yourself and your child in a way that allows you to feel comfortable. Put the best effort towards paying attention to your child's tooth decay. If you have a dentist with whom you already have a relationship, then in the case of an emergency or urgent need, you will at least not have the added stress of finding a dentist. There are some dentists who are self-confident. They trust themselves and as a result they do not pressure the parents to perform needless dental surgery. They do not rush you into decisions or manipulate you to submit to drastic dental procedures. Dentists can help support the monitoring of tooth decay to make sure it does not progress. This will help some parents feel better. I urge you to be cautious here, as many dentists offer harmful advice and treatments.

First, I want to acknowledge what a stressful and terrible situation many parents face with their dentist. Many mothers have contacted me, upset by the violent and aggressive attitudes that dentists have concerning treatment for children. Not all dentists are like this, but it seems very common.

In a majority of cases dentists whose focus is not on giving complete dental surgery for children will give you much better treatment than those whose income is based on performing surgery under general anesthesia. Generally these are dentists who do not specialize in children's dentistry.

## Topical Care for Infants' and Children's Teeth

Toothbrushes, tooth pastes, sealants, and other facsimiles do little to prevent or cure tooth decay in children. You will want to use natural tooth cleaning as discussed in chapter eight about dentistry. Since the brushing movements of children can be inaccurate, they are likely to brush into their gums, and jam plaque up into the gum line. A soft bristle brush or a cloth and teaching your child how to gently clean the gums and soft tissues of the mouth with a brush seem to be the best ideas for cleaning children's mouths.

# A Little More about Early Childhood Tooth Decay

**White spot lesions** are the white areas which are not always tooth decay, but are usually the first visually detectable signs of it. They are smooth patches or markings that usually form along the gum line.

Children who experience successful treatment through nutrition have no tooth pain and no tooth or gum infections. The child also has no sensitivity to hot or cold foods nor a fear of biting into things. The white spots may fade away and the decayed tooth material in the cavities turns from sticky or soft, with a light brown color, to dark and hard. The edges of the cavities will stop spreading or the spread will be minimal. The child's gum tissue will be firm and pink. The remineralized dentin (the healthy middle layer of the tooth below the enamel) on any decayed teeth will have a yellow or white tinge, and the appearance can be glassy.

> **Knocked-out baby tooth.** Do not perform a root canal on the tooth. Reimplant it as soon as possible and use homeopathic remedies like arnica and hypericum.[309]

> **Chipped teeth.** A small chip probably does not need to be repaired. A more severe chip can be repaired with bonding materials. If the nerve is exposed, do not give your child a root canal. Use homeopathic calendula and have a good dentist use a dental base and composite materials to seal it.[310]

## Homeopathic Cell Salts

Homeopathic cell salts, or tissue salts help improve absorption and utilization of minerals at the cellular level. They can help balance digestion and remove toxins from the body. Working with a practitioner who can help you use homeopathic cell salts can be a beneficial way to help heal your child's cavities by improving nutrient absorption. Likewise, finding support using food-based dietary supplements like Standard Process™ can also aid in healing children's cavities by correcting nutrient deficiencies.

## Pregnancy and Cavities

During pregnancy and breastfeeding, the nutritional burden on the mother's body is much higher than usual because she is eating for two people. While the diet of a mother before pregnancy may have been adequate, with the higher nutritional demands of pregnancy and lactation the former diet may not provide enough nutrients, and tooth decay can be the result. Pregnancy is also a time when extra hormones (such as estrogen) are being released. At this time of increased physical demands, minerals can easily be pulled from the bones and previous imbalances

**Tuscarora Native American mother from New York who ate a modernized diet.**

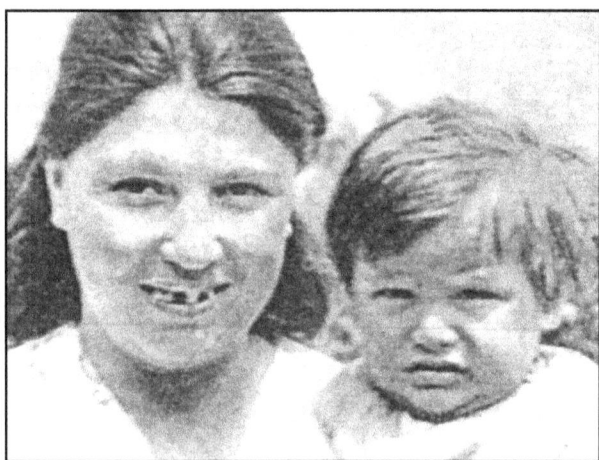

*Copyright © Price-Pottenger Nutrition Foundation, www.ppnf.org*

*A typical mother was studied at her home. She had four children. Her teeth were ravaged by dental caries. She was strictly modern, for she had gold inlays in some of her teeth. The roots of the missing teeth had not been extracted. Twenty of her teeth had active dental caries. Her little girl, aged four, already had twelve badly decayed teeth.*[311]

**Mother on native diet of seafood with no tooth decay.**

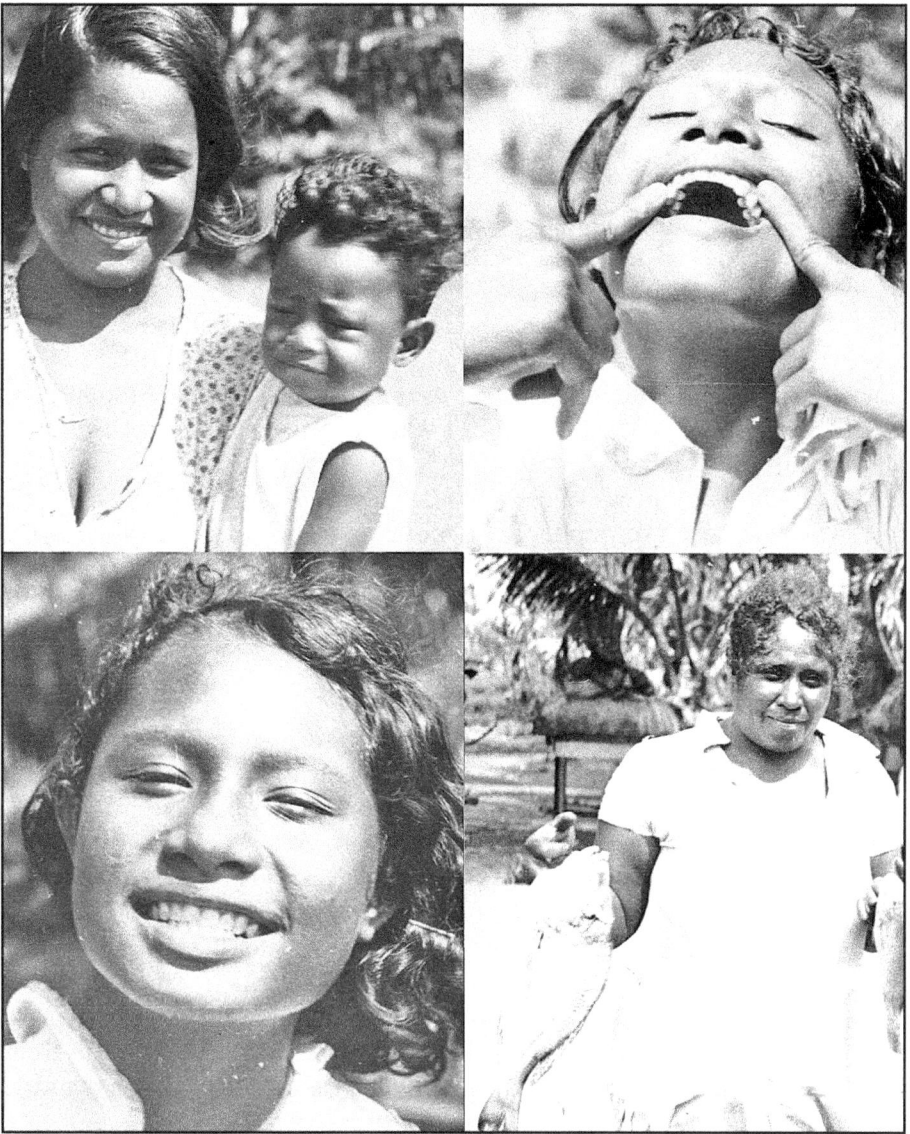

*Copyright © Price-Pottenger Nutrition Foundation, www.ppnf.org*

*These pictures tell an interesting story. The grandmother shown in the lower right knew the importance of seafood for her children and grandchildren and did the fishing herself. Note the beautiful teeth and well formed faces of her daughters.[312] The young mother above is free from tooth decay.*

can become exaggerated. This can also contribute to tooth decay. A diet which includes fat-soluble vitamins will help to balance this condition. Healing cavities with nutrition during pregnancy or lactation provides an added health benefit: your child will be more robust and healthy from the extra nutrients you provide. Your birth recovery will also be enhanced because your body will have a greater storage of nutrients to utilize during and after the birth. Your life as a new mother will—one hopes—proceed more smoothly, because you will have more energy to care for the new baby. Soups are particularly nourishing for pregnancy and after birth.

Tooth decay often occurs during pregnancy because the mother's body is engaged in the borrowing process. The borrowing process is illustrated in next photo. You can compare two mothers, one with widespread tooth decay and the other with none. The difference is that the mother with extensive tooth decay consumed a modern diet, and the mother without tooth decay ate her native diet which in this case was rich in sea food.

When your body does not receive enough nutrients during pregnancy, it will borrow minerals from your teeth. It is important to emphasize that this problem is usually dietary and there is nothing inherently wrong with the woman herself. Her body is simply responding to a set of particular circumstances.

## *Breastfeeding and Cavities*

Breast milk provides protection from cavities, so night-time nursing does not cause or promote tooth decay. The claim that night-time nursing causes tooth decay is simply anti-breastfeeding propaganda and is not scientifically based.

The American Academy of Pediatric Dentistry (AAPD) presents contradictory positions on breastfeeding. They support both day and night breastfeeding in their official policy, stating that "breast-feeding ensures the best possible health as well as the best development and psychosocial outcomes for the infant."[313] Their recommendation formerly advised avoidance of on-cue night time breastfeeding after the first teeth erupt, but that no longer is the official policy. The AAPD policy *suggests* that mothers not breastfeed a child on cue after the first teeth erupt to reduce cavities, morning and night for all children.[314] I disagree with this idea. This concept is also not supported by studies provided on their own website. In fact, AAPD published a press release about a study which states, "breast milk prohibits acid and bacterial growth in the mouth."[315] This would imply that you would want to breastfeed your child to prevent cavities. An interesting note on this report is that breast milk by itself was not shown to contribute to cavities, but when breastfeeding was alternated with sweet foods it did promote cavities. This sounds a lot like what W.D. Miller reported in 1883 when he stated that a healthy tooth resists acid or other substances, but that a weak tooth succumbs quickly to tooth decay. In the case of a child with very weak teeth from too much sugar or grain bran and germ, it might appear that breast milk promoted cavities since anything with any sweetness at all would promote cavities at that point.

Night-time nursing helps protect against tooth decay. Children under the age of three who grow during the night need breast milk on cue to provide their bodies with the nutrients they need for health. Children over the age of three may need less breastfeeding at night, but still some to help them sleep well. Many children breastfeed at night and do not have cavities. Studies do not show a link between long-term breastfeeding and a higher number of cavities.[316] It is important to be clear about this. Commercial formulas usually have sugar added. The use of these formulas or the use of fruit juices, for nighttime bottle feeding, will increase the likelihood of tooth decay. Breast milk is the best food there is for your baby. If your child is experiencing decay, then one must examine what other foods in the diet may be causing this decay, and not condemn breast milk or avoid breastfeeding.

Many breastfed children have tooth decay even though breast milk protects against bacteria in the mouth.[317] How, then, can we say that tooth decay is caused by bacteria, when children constantly have naturally antibacterial milk in their mouths to retard the decay?

Recently I've learned of an important and overlooked factor regarding breast-feeding and cavities. Some young children who have cavities are being breastfed regularly over an extended period of time. We know that cavities occur when the body chemistry is out of balance. How could it be that breast milk would seem to unbalance a child's body chemistry, considering it is the ideal food? As the child feeds for an extended period on the same breast, the milk becomes thicker, and the fat content increases. If the mother mistakenly and consistently feeds her child too much of the foremilk, which is sweet and lower in fat, then this could hypothetically create a body chemistry imbalance over time. Other factors, such as the mother not drinking enough fluids, or the intake of other inharmonious substances, can also cause imbalances in the breast milk. A nourished child drinks plenty of hind milk, which is higher in fat. The baby will digest this milk more slowly, due to its higher fat content. If there is stress associated with breastfeed-ing, or the mother doesn't allow full breast feeding sessions, then again the child may be receiving excessive amounts of the sweeter fore milk, which may contribute to the formation of cavities. Attentive breastfeeding techniques will give your child the best potential to be free of cavities.

I know breastfeeding is a delicate subject. I support breastfeeding children on cue for long extended periods, even for 4–7 years. I discuss this in greater detail in my book on early childhood and health, *Healing Our Children*, **www. healingourchildren.org** If a parent is not careful then breast milk can become an incomplete food for her child. As a child ages she needs more and more nutrients from food. The amount of nutrients from food and from breast milk need to be balanced based upon the age and physical development of the child. Weaning is not the answer, but rather simply finding the balance of enough breastfeeding and enough supplemental solid foods.

Finally, having the highest amount of vitamins and minerals possible in the breast milk will help your young child grow strong and prosper. The breastfeeding mother of a child with significant tooth decay should supplement her diet with many of the special foods described in this book, including high vitamin butter and liver or cod liver oil, along with food-source vitamin C and adequate calcium.

## Close Your Baby's Mouth at Night

When I first read about this principle it sounded peculiar to me. Of course our bodies are designed to primarily breathe through our noses. Otherwise why do we have noses? Yet some children and adults are primarily mouth breathers. The syndrome of breathing through the mouth when asleep is associated with a smaller jaw size, bed wetting, ear infections, heart disease, hypertension, and snoring.[318] How your child's jaw grows and develops may even be connected to how he breathes at night. George Catlin's book, *Shut Your Mouth and Save Your Life*, describes practices of Native Americans with whom Mr. Catlin lived during the mid 1800s. Mothers always made sure that from birth, their children slept with their mouths closed. An open mouth at night can, among other things, affect the substance P level in the body and affect the trigeminal nerve which could possibly have adverse repercussions on the child's growth and physical development. After you breastfeed at night, make sure your baby's mouth is removed from the nipple and closed so that she is breathing through her nose.

## Fathers and Tooth Decay

I have talked with many mothers who are struggling with their child's tooth decay. The problem seems to be related to the relationship between the father and the mother, or between the father and the child. Single moms can easily feel particularly stressed because they do not have the support that they need to take care of their child. Many mothers also have to deal with fathers who do not care as much as is necessary to provide their child with healthy food. There appears to be a connection between the lack of nourishment in a child, and the absence—either physically or emotionally—of the father, since part of the father's primal role is to provide nourishment for the family. For couples who are together, fathers of children with cavities need to play an active role in supporting the mother. For single mothers, notice how the absence of the father is affecting you.

## *Final Thoughts on Remineralizing Your Child's Tooth Decay*

Dental treatments only address the symptoms of tooth decay. They were not designed for children, nor are these treatments proven to work for them. Because tooth decay is not caused by bacteria, dental treatments cannot prevent tooth decay. Children grow rapidly in their early years and, with these high demands for nutrients, their bodies can easily become depleted. We need to feed them well so they are strong and feel happy.

We do not have to be victims of tooth decay. The dietary guidelines I have suggested, when closely followed, are a powerful tool for preventing and halting tooth decay. In the wake of these dysfunctional treatments for tooth decay, there lies a simple and profound method to dramatically improve the health of your children: good nutrition.

Since about 82% of children's decayed primary teeth fall out without them experiencing any symptoms and without any sort of nutritional treatment, imagine what the results would be with specially reinforced nutrition to prevent against infection and remineralize the tooth. Even with successful nutritional treatments, the teeth might still decay a bit for a while, and some may not look very attractive. Even if one or two baby teeth do not make it to their full life, changing your child's diet will make a lasting impact on his health for the rest of his life and help form healthy adult teeth.

Your child's dental health is in your hands. Reclaim responsibility for your children's dental health!

# About the Author

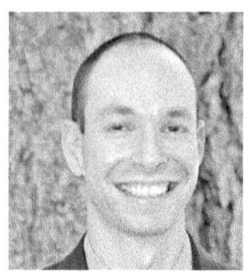

**Ramiel Nagel** is a father who resides in Los Gatos, California. Ramiel became interested in natural health when he discovered that his daughter was suffering from tooth decay. His background of study includes emotional health care, hatha yoga and bhakti yoga of devotion.

Ramiel earned a B.A. in Legal Studies from the University of California at Santa Cruz. He feels compelled to bring the knowledge contained in this book to the world so that other people can be healthier and happier. The work is done in the spirit of service to all.

His health websites include:

**www.yourreturn.org**

**www.curetoothdecay.com**

**www.healingourchildren.org**

**www.preconceptionhealth.org**

# How to Order Additional Copies of Cure Tooth Decay

Visit my website for easy online ordering:

**www.curetoothdecay.com**

For bulk purchases please e-mail Golden Child Publishing
orders@goldenchildpublishing.com

# Endnotes

1 American Academy of Biologic Dentistry, May 1987 Iatrogenic Damage Due To High Speed Drilling by Ralph Turk, DDS, Germany

2 Brown, E.H. & Hansen, R.T. The Key to Ultimate Health. Fullerton: Advanced Health Research Publishing; 1998:32-33.

3 Hussain, Sharmila. "Chapter 15." Textbook of Dental Materials. New Delhi: Jaypee Brothers Medical, 2004. 258. Print.

4 Ring ME (2005). "Founders of a profession: the original subscribers to the first dental journal in the world". The Journal of the American College of Dentists 72 (2): 20–5.

5 Huggins, H. A. DDS It's All In Your Head. Garden City Park, New York: Avery; 1993:61.

6 Breiner, M. DDS Whole-Body Dentistry. Fairfield: Quantum Health Press; 1999:59-60.

7 Huggins, H. A. DR It's All In Your Head. Garden City Park, New York: Avery; 1993:43-52.

8 Breiner, M. DDS Whole-Body Dentistry. Fairfield: Quantum Health Press; 1999:137-138.

9 Ibid., 79.

10 Ibid., 78.

11 Jeans, P.C. A Survey of Literature of Dental Caries: Washington, D.C.: National Academy of Sciences; 1952:251.

12 Ibid., 251.

13 Tooth Decay, FAQ, American Dental Association. Available at: http://www.ada.org/public/topics/decay_faq. asp.

14 Why is Sugar in Food, Sugar Association. Available At:: http://www.sugar.org/consumers/ sweet_by_nature. asp?id=279.

15 Osmotic pressure and bacteria – Science Encyclopedia http://science.jrank.org/pages/714/Bacteria.html

16 CDS Review. "NIDCR Studies Oral Biofilms". No author listed. January/February 2005, page 60.

17 Howe, P. DDS. Further Studies of the Effect of Diet Upon the Teeth and Bones Journal of the American Dental Association, 1923: 201

18 Larmas, M., J Dent Res 82:253 (2003)

19 Schatz, A. The New York State Dental Journal: Vol. 38, No. 3: 285-295: May, 1972

20 Roggenkamp, Clyde L., and John Leonora. "Foreward." Dentinal Fluid Transport : Publications of Drs. Ralph Steinman and John Leonora. Loma Linda, CA: Loma Linda University School of Dentistry, 2004. XIV. Print.

21 Ibid., VI.

22 Surveillance for Dental Caries, Dental Sealants, Tooth Retention, Edentulism, and Enamel Fluorosis—United States, 1988–1994 and 1999–2002. Centers for Disease Control and Prevention (CDC), Available at: http://www. cdc. gov/MMWR/preview/mmwrhtml/ ss5403a1.htm

23 National Health and Nutrition Examination Survey, 1999-2002. NationalCenter for Health Statistics, CDC. Available at: www.cdc.gov/ nccdphp/publications/aag/ pdf/oh.pdf.

24 Trends in Oral Health Status: United States, 1988-1994 and 1999-2004. Series 11, Number 248. 104 pp. (PHS) 2007-1698.

25 Price, W. A. Journal of the American Dental Association, 1936: 888.

26 Ibid., 26.

27 Ibid.

28 Ibid.

29 Ibid., 35.

30 Ibid., 39.

31 Ibid., 27.

32 Price, "Why Dental Caries with Modern Civilizations? V. An Interpretation of Field Studies Previously Reported," 278.

33 Figures have been rounded up for simplicity

34 op. cit., p. 27.

35 Price, "Why Dental Caries with Modern Civilizations? V. An Interpretation of Field Studies Previously Reported," 278.

36 Ibid., 35.

37 op. cit., p. 38.

38 Ibid., 45.

39 Ibid., 44.

40 Ibid.

41 Ibid., 49.

42 Ibid.

43 Ibid.

44 Ibid. 50.

45 Ibid 49.

46 Ibid., 55-57.

47 Price, W.A. Dental Digest, Figure Ten.

48 Price, W. A. Nutrition and Physical Degeneration 6th Edition. La Mesa: Price-Pottenger Nutrition Foundation; 2004: op. cit., p. 441.

49 op. cit., p. 171.

50 op. cit., p. 173.

51 op. cit., p. 174.

52 Ibid., 186.

53 Fallon, S. and Enig, M. Australian Aborigines— Living Off the Fat of the Land, Available At: http://www. westonaprice.org/traditional_diets/australian_aborigines.html

54 Price, W. A. Nutrition and Physical Degeneration 6th Edition. La Mesa: Price-Pottenger Nutrition Foundation; 2004: op. cit., p. 174.

55 op. cit., p. 275-276.

56 Price, W. A. Nutrition and Physical Degeneration 6th Edition. La Mesa: Price-Pottenger Nutrition Foundation; 2004:415.

57 Price, Weston A. "Field Studies among Some African Tribes on the Relation of Their Nutrition to the Incidence of Dental Caries and Dental Arch Deformities" Journal. A.D.A. 23:888, May 1936.

58 SUPPLEMENTARY DATA TABLES, USDA's 1994-96 Continuing Survey of Food Intakes by Individuals, Table Set 12, US Department of Agriculture, Agricultural Research Service, Available at: http://www.ars.usda.gov/ SP2UserFiles/Place/12355000/pdf/Supp.PDF.

59 Price, W. A. Nutrition and Physical Degeneration 6th Edition. La Mesa: Price-Pottenger Nutrition Foundation; 2004:295.

60 Ibid., 432.

61 Price, W. A. Nutrition and Physical Degeneration 8th Edition. La Mesa: Price-Pottenger Nutrition Foundation; 2008:391-392.

62 Price, W. A. *Nutrition and Physical Degeneration 6th Edition.* La Mesa: Price-Pottenger Nutrition Foundation; 2004:290.

63 Ibid., 295.

64 Ibid., 273.

65 Ibid., 274.

66 Ibid., 488.

67 Page, M. Abrams, L. Your Body is Your Best Doctor. New Canaan: Keats Publishing Inc.; 1972:188.

68 Page, M. Abrams, L. Your Body is Your Best Doctor. New Canaan: Keats Publishing Inc.; 1972:196.

69 Forbes, R. The Hormone Mess And How To Fix It. 2004: 7.

70 Page, M. Abrams, L. Your Body is Your Best Doctor. New Canaan: Keats Publishing Inc.;1972:196.

71 Ibid., 23.

72 Cook, Douglas DDS "Rescued by My Dentist.": 27.

73 Berggren G. ,Brannstrom M., "The Rate of Flow in Dentinal Tubules Due to Capillary Attraction." J Dent Res.1965; 44: 307-456.

74 Ten Cate AR. Oral Histology: Development, Structure and Function. Mosby, St. Louis, Boston, Toronto 1998; Chapters 5, 9, 10, 11 and 18.

75 Roggenkamp, Clyde L., and John Leonora. "Foreward." Dentinal Fluid Transport : Publications of Drs. Ralph Steinman and John Leonora. Loma Linda, CA: Loma Linda University School of Dentistry, 2004. IX. Print.

76 Huggins, Hal A., DDS. Why Raise Ugly Kids. Arlington House Publishers, Westport, CT, Copyright 1981, ISBNO-87000-507-3, pages 143-149.

77 Forbes, R. The Hormone Mess and How to Fix It. 2004: 12.

78 Ravnskov MD, Uffe. "The Cholesterol Myths." Cholesterol Myths. 7 Sept. 2006. Web. 16 Aug. 2010. <http://www.ravnskov.nu/cholesterol.htm>.

79 Ibid.

80 http://www.westonaprice.org/abcs-of-nutrition/173.html

81 Mellanby, E. Relation of Diet to Health and Disease. The British Medical Journal 677, April 12, 1930.

82 Masterjohn, Chris. "On the Trail of the Elusive X-Factor: A Sixty-Two-Year-Old Mystery Finally Solved." The Weston A. Price Foundation. 13 Feb. 2008. Web. 16 Aug. 2010. <http://www.westonaprice.org/abcs-of-nutrition/175-x-factor-is-vitamin-k2.html>.

83 Masterjohn, Chris. "From Seafood to Sunshine: A New Understanding of Vitamin D Safety." The Weston A. Price Foundation. Dec. 2006. Web. 15 Aug. 2010. <http://www.westonaprice.org/abcs-of-nutrition/173.html>.

84 Sullivan, Krispin. "The Miracle of Vitamin D." The Weston A. Price Foundation. Dec. 2000. Web. 16 Aug. 2010. <http://www.westonaprice.org/ abcs-of-nutrition/168.html>.

85 Wetzel, Dave. "Part 2, Deeper Discussion; Why FCLO and High Vitamin Butter Oil." Green Pasture Products. July 2010. Web. 16 Aug. 2010. <http://www.greenpasture.org/community/?q=node/271>.

86 Ibid.

87 Mellanby, May. "THE AETIOLOGY OF DENTAL CARIES." British Medical Journal (1932): 749-51. Print.

88 Masterjohn, Chris. "Vitamin A On Trial: Does Vitamin A Cause Osteoporosis?" The Weston A. Price Foundation. 1 Aug. 2006. Web. 22 Aug. 2010. <http://www.westonaprice.org/abcs-of-nutrition/172-vitamin-a-on-trial.html>.

89 Ibid.

90 Ibid.

91 Vitamin A figures from http://www.nutritiondata.com which is extracted from USDA government data on vitamin contents of food.

92 Wetzel, Dave. "Part 2, Deeper Discussion; Why FCLO and High Vitamin Butter Oil Products." Green Pasture Products. July 2010. Web. 16 Aug. 2010. <http://www.greenpasture.org/community/?q=node/271>.

93 Ibid.

94 Fallon, Sally, and Mary Enig. "Cod Liver Oil Basics and Recommendations." The Weston A. Price Foundation. 8 Feb. 2009. Web. 23 Aug. 2010. <http://www.westonaprice.org/cod-liver-oil/238.html>.

95 Masterjohn, Chris. "Vitamin A On Trial: Does Vitamin A Cause Osteoporosis?" The Weston A. Price Foundation. 1 Aug. 2006. Web. 22 Aug. 2010. <http://www.westonaprice.org/abcs-of-nutrition/172-vitamin-a-on-trial.html>.

96 Price, W. A. Nutrition and Physical Degeneration 8th Edition. La Mesa: Price-Pottenger Nutrition Foundation; 2008:269.

97 Wetzel, David. "Cod Liver Oil Manufacturing." The Weston A. Price Foundation. 28 Feb. 2006. Web. 22 Aug. 2010. <http://www.westonaprice. org/cod-liver-oil/183-clo-manufacturing.html>.

98 Fallon, Sally, and Mary Enig. "Cod Liver Oil Basics and Recommendations." The Weston A. Price Foundation. 8 Feb. 2008. Web. 23 Aug. 2010. <http://www.westonaprice.org/cod-liver-oil/238.html#brands>.

99 Price, W. A. Nutrition and Physical Degeneration 6th Edition. La Mesa: Price-Pottenger Nutrition Foundation; 2004:26.

100 Price, W. A. *Nutrition and Physical Degeneration* 8th Edition. La Mesa: Price-Pottenger Nutrition Foundation; 2008:385.

101 Ibid., 386.

102 Wetzel, Dave. "Plant Stem Cells." Green Pasture Products. 9 Mar. 2010. Web. 22 Aug. 2010. <http://www.greenpasture.org/community/?q=node/231>.

103 Price, W. A. *Nutrition and Physical Degeneration* 8th Edition. La Mesa: Price-Pottenger Nutrition Foundation; 2008:391.

104 Price, "Why Dental Caries with Modern Civilizations?" XI. New Light on Loss of Immunity to Some Degenerative Processes Including Dental Caries," 243.

105 Price, "Why Dental Caries with Modern Civilizations? XI. New Light on Loss of Immunity to Some Degenerative Processes Including Dental Caries," 243.

106 Wetzel, Dave. "Update on Cod Liver Oil Manufacture." The Weston A. Price Foundation. 30 Apr. 2009. Web. 23 Aug. 2010. <http://www.westonaprice.org/cod-liver-oil/1602-update-on-cod-liver-oil-manufacture.html>.

107 Heard, George W. "Chapter 17." *Man versus Toothache.* Milwaukee: Lee Foundation for Nutritional Research, 1952. Print.

108  Ibid., Chapter 9.

109  Ibid., Chapter 28.

110  McAfee, Mark. "The Fifteen Things That Pasteurization Kills." *Wise Traditions* Summer (2010): 82. Print.

111  Ibid.

112  Huggins, Hal A.. *It's All in Your Head: The Link Between Mercury Amalgams and Illness.* 1 ed. New York: Avery Publishing, 1993. Print:155.

113  USDA food nutrient database accessed at www.nutritiondata.com

114  Page, Melvin E., and H. Leon Abrams. *Your Body Is Your Best Doctor!* New Canaan, CT: Keats Pub., 1972. 129. Print.

115  Price, W. A. *Nutrition and Physical Degeneration* 8th Edition. La Mesa: Price-Pottenger Nutrition Foundation; 2008:29.

116  Ibid., 113-114.

117  Page, Melvin E., and H. Leon. Abrams. *Health vs Disease, a Revolution in Medical Thinking.* St. Petersburg, FL: Page Foundation, 1960. 57. Print.

118  Tooth Decay, Pregnancy FAQ, American Dental Association. Available at: http://www.ada.org/ public/topics/pregnancy_faq.asp

119  Huggins, Hal A.. *It's All in Your Head: The Link Between Mercury Amalgams and Illness.* 1 ed. New York: Avery Publishing, 1993. Print:156.

120  Burt, Brian A. "The use of sorbitol- and xylitol-sweetened chewing gum in caries control." *Journal of the American Dental Association* Vol 137, No 2, 190–196. Jan. 2008 <http://jada.ada.org/ cgi/content/abstract/137/2/190>.

121  "Artificial Sweeteners Symptoms, Causes, Treatment— Are There Any Safety Concerns with Sugar Alcohols on MedicineNet." Web. 01 Sept. 2010. <http://www.medicinenet.com/ artificial_sweeteners/page4.htm>.

122  Eyre, Charlotte. "Sugar-free Gum Poisonous for Pets." Confectionery News—News on Confectionery. 24 June 2007. Web. 31 Aug. 2010. <http://www.confectionerynews.com/Markets/Sugar-free-gum-poisonous-for-pets>.

123  1.Dehmel KH and others. Absorption of xylitol. Int. Symp on metabolism, physiololgy and clinical use of pentoses and pentitols. Hakone, Japan, 1967, 177-181, Ed. Horecker. www.inchem.org/ documents/jecfa/jecmono/v12je22.htm

124  Heaney, Anthony. "UCLA's Jonsson Comprehensive Cancer Center : In the News : Pancreatic Cancers Use Fructose, Common in a Western Diet, to Fuel Growth." UCLA's Jonsson Comprehensive Cancer Center : Cancer Treatment and Research. 3 Aug. 2010. Web. 01 Sept. 2010. <http://www.cancer.ucla.edu/ Index.aspx? page=6 44&recordid=385&returnURL=/index.aspx>.

125  Page, Melvin E., and H. Leon Abrams. *Your Body Is Your Best Doctor!* New Canaan, CT: Keats Pub., 1972. 184. Print.

126  Davidson, Lena. "Iron Bioavailablity from Weaning Foods: The Effect of Phytic Acid" Macronutrient Interactions: Impact on Child Health and Nutrition by US Agency for International Development Food and Agricultural Organization of the United Nations. 1996:23.

127  Johnson DDS, Clarke. "Epidemiology of Dental Disease." *University of Illinois at Chicago—UIC.* N.p., n.d. Web. 13 Sept. 2010

128  Mellanby, E. Relation of Diet to Health and Disease. *The British Medical Journal* 677, April 12, 1930.

129  Barnett Cohen and Lafayette B. Mendel. Experimental Scurvy of the Guinea Pig in Relation to The Diet, *J. Biol. Chem.* 1918 35: 425-453.

130  Ibid., 449.

131  Iron absorption in man: ascrobic acid and dose-depended inhibition. *American Journal of Clinical Nutrition.* Jan 1989. 49(1):140-144.

132  Mellanby, Edward J. The Rickets-Producing and Anti-Calcifying Action of Phytate Physiol. (1949) 109, 488-533 547.593:6I2.751.1

133  McCollum, Elmer Verner. *The New Knowledge of Nutrition.* New York: Macmillan, 1918. 312. Print. (Professor of Chemical Hygiene, John Hopkins University)

134  Ibid., 316.

135  Ibid., 324.

136  Mellanby, Edward J. The Rickets-Producing and Anti-Calcifying Action of Phytate *Physiol.* (1949) 109, 488-533 547.593:6I2.751.1

137  On Cases Described as "Acute Rickets," which are probably a combination of Scurvy and Rickets, the Scurvy being an essential, and the rickets a variable, element *Med Chir* Trans. 1883; 66: 159–220.1.

138  Sherlock, Paul, Rothschild, E. Scurvy Produced by a Zen Macrobiotic Diet *JAMA,* March 13, 1967. Vol 199, No 11

139  Mellanby, May, and Lee Pattison. "THE INFLUENCE OF A CEREAL-FREE DIET RICH IN VITAMIN D AND CALCIUM ON DENTAL CARIES IN CHILDREN." *British Medical Journal* (1932): 507-12. Print.

140  Ibid.

141  Mellanby, Edward. "The Relation of Diet to Health and Disease." *British Medical Journal* (1930): 677-81. Print.

142  *J. Physiol.* (1942) 101, 44-8 612.015.31 Mineral Metabolism of Healthy Adults on White and Brown Bread Dietaries.

143  Mellanby, Edward, and D. C. Harrison. "Phytic Acid and the Rickets-producing Action of Cereals." *Biochemical Journal* (1939): 1660-674. Print.

144  Mellanby, Edward. "The Rickets-Producing an dAnti-Calcifying Action of Phytate." *J. Physiol.* (1949) 109, 488-533

145  Davidson, Lena. "Iron Bioavailablity from Weaning Foods: The Effect of Phytic Acid" Macronutrient Interactions: Impact on Child Health and Nutrition by US Agency for International Development Food and Agricultural Organization of the United Nations. 1996:22.

146  Johansen K and others. Degradation of phytate in soaked diets for pigs. Department of Animal Health, Welfare and Nutrition, Danish Institute of Agricultural Sciences, Research Centre Foulum, Tjele, Denmark.

147  Tannenbaum and others. *Vitamins and Minerals in Food Chemistry,* 2nd edition. OR Fennema, ed. Marcel Dekker, Inc., New York, 1985, p 445.

148  Ibid.

149  Singh M and Krikorian D. Inhibition of trypsin activity in vitro by phytate. *Journal of Agricultural and Food Chemistry* 1982 30(4):799-800.

150  Ibid.

151  "Fermented cereals a global perspective. Table of contents.." *FAO: FAO Home.* N.p., n.d. Web. 13 Sept. 2010. <http://www.fao.org/docrep/ x2184E/x2184E00.htm >

152  Ibid.

153  Ibid.

154  Daniel, Kaayla. "Plants Bite Back." *Wise Traditions* 11.1: 18-26. Print.

155  Denny, Paul. et al. Novel Caries Risk Test» DOI: 10.1196/ annals.1384.009

156  Antinutritional content of developed weaning foods as affected by domestic processing. *Food Chemistry.* 1993 47(4):333-336.

157  I. EGLI, L. DAVIDSSON, M.A. JUILLERAT, D. BAR- CLAY, R.F. HURRELL. "The Influence of Soaking and Germination on the Phytase Activity and Phytic Acid Content of Grains and Seeds Potentially Useful for Complementary Feeding." *Sensory and nutritive quali- ties of food* 67.9 (2002): 3484-3488. Print.

158  Ibid.

159  Silvia Valencia, Ulf Svanberg, Ann-Sofie Sandberg, Jenny Ruales Processing of quinoa (Chenopodium quinoa, Willd): effects on in vitro iron availability and phytate hydrolysis *International Journal of Food Sciences and Nutrition.* 1999, Vol. 50, No. 3 , Pages 203-211

160  Fazli Manan, Tajammal Hussain, Inteaz Alli and Parvez Iqbal. "Effect of cooking on phytic acid content and nutritive value of Pakistani peas and lentils." *Food Chem- istry* Volume 23, Issue 2, 1987, Pages 81-87.

161  *Food Chemistry* 1993. 47(4)333-336.

162  SAMUEL KON, DAVID W. SANSHUCK PHYTATE CONTENT AND ITS EFFECT ON COOKING QUALITY OF BEANS. *Journal of Food Processing and Preservation.* Volume 5, Issue 3, pages 169–178, September 1981.

163  "Fermented cereals a global perspective. Table of con- tents.." *FAO: FAO Home.* N.p., n.d. Web. 13 Sept. 2010. <http://www.fao.org/docrep/ x2184E/x2184E00.htm >

164  Rubel, William. "Rye Bread from France : Pain Bouilli." William Rubel, Author and Cook Specializing in Tra- ditional Cuisines. Web. 4 Sept. 2010. <http://www. williamrubel.com/artisanbread/examples/ryebread/ rye-bread-from-france-pain-bouilli>. Further reading Marcel Maget's Le pain anniversaire a Vilard d'Arene en Oisans

165  Ibid.

166  Czapp, Katherine. "The Good Scots Diet." The Weston A. Price Foundation. 1 May 2009. Web. 04 Sept. 2010. <http://www.westonaprice.org/traditional-diets/1605. html>.

167  Conversation on "Basmati Rice." IndiaDivine. Web. 07 Sept. 2010. <http://www.indiadivine.org/ audarya/ ayurveda-health-wellbeing/902739-basmati-rice.html>.

168  Trinidad P. Trinidada; Aida C. Mallillina; Rosario S. Saguma; Dave P. Brionesa; Rosario R. Encaboa; Bien- venido O. Julianob . "Iron absorption from brown rice/ brown rice-based meal and milled rice/milled rice-based meal." *International Journal of Food Sciences and Nutri- tion*, Volume 60, Issue 8 December 2009 , pages 688- 693.

169  Rice and iron absorption in man. European Journal of Clinical Nutrition. July 1990. 44(7):489-497.

170  "Fermented cereals a global perspective. Table of con- tents.." *FAO: FAO Home.* N.p., n.d. Web. 13 Sept. 2010. <http://www.fao.org/docrep/ x2184E/x2184E00.htm >

171  McKenzie-Parnell JM and Davies NT. Destruction of Phytic Acid During Home Breadmaking. *Food Chemistry* 1986 22:181–192.

172  CCVIII. PHYTIC ACID AND THE RICKETSPRODUC- ING ACTION OF CEREALS BY DOUGLAS CREESE HARRISON AD EDWARD MELLANBY From the Field Laboratory, University of Sheffield, and the Department of Biochemistry, Queen's University, Belfast (Received 11 August 1939)

173  Mellanby, Edward J. The Rickets-Producing and Anti- Calcifying Action of Phytate *J.Physiol.* (1949) 109, 488- 533 547.593:612.751.1

174  Ologhobo AD and Fetuga BL. Distribution of Phospho- rus and Phytate in Some Nigerian Varieties of Legumes and some Effects of Processing. *Journal of Food Science* 1984 Volume 49.

175  Fallon, Sally, and Mary G. Enig. *Nourishing Traditions: the Cookbook That Challenges Politically Correct Nutrition and the Diet Dictocrats.* Washington, DC: New Trends Pub., 2001. 468-69. Print.

176  Macfarlane, Bezwoda, Bothwell, Baynes, Bothwell, MacPhail, Lamparelli, Mayet. "inhibitory effect of nuts on iron absorption." *The American Journal of Clinical Nutrition* 47 (1988): 270-274. Print.

177  Ibid.

178  Ibid.

179  N. R. Reddy, Shridhar K. Sathe. *Food Phytates.* 1 ed. Boca Raton, FL: CRC Press, 2001. Print.

180  McGlone, John, and Wilson G. Pond. *Pig Production: Biological Principles and Applications.* 1 ed. Albany: Del- mar Cengage Learning, 2002. Print.

181  Lonnerdal and Dewey. *Micronutrient Interactions US Agency of International Development* / Food and Agricul- ture Organization of the United Nations: 1995.

182  Masterjohn, Chris. "Vitamin A On Trial: Does Vitamin A Cause Osteoporosis?" The Weston A. Price Foundation. 1 Aug. 2006. Web. 22 Aug. 2010. <http://www.westonaprice. org/abcs-of-nutrition/172-vitamin-a-on-trial.html>.

183  Huggins, Hal A.. *It's All in Your Head: The Link Between Mercury Amalgams and Illness.* 1 ed. New York: Avery Publishing, 1993. Print:147.

184  Bieler, H. *Food is Your Best Medicine.* New York: Vintage Books, 1965: 202.

185  "Soy Alert!" The Weston A. Price Foundation. Web. 02 Sept. 2010. <http://www.westonaprice. org/soy-alert. html>.

186  Smith, Garret. "Nightshades:oblems from These Popular Foods Exposed to the Light of Day." *Wise Traditions* 11.1 (2010): 48-54. Print.

187  Brown, Ellen Hodgson., and Richard T. Hansen. The Key to Ultimate Health: Researchers Worldwide Are Concluding That a Vital Key to Wellness Have Been Overlooked—and It's Right under Your Nose! Fullerton, CA: *Advanced Health Research Pub.*, 1998:174. Print.

188  Brian Q. Phillippya, Mengshi Linb, Barbara Rascob. Analysis of phytate in raw and cooked potatoes. *Journal of Food Composition and Analysis* 17 (2004) 217–226.

189  BRIAN Q. PHILLIPPY,JOHN M. BLAND, AND TER- ENCE J. EVENS, Ion Chromatography of Phytate in Roots and Tubers. *J. Agric. Food Chem.* 2003, 51, 350- 353.

190  Ibid.

191  Richard A. Fenske, John C. Kissel, Chensheng Lu, David A. Kalman, Nancy J. Simcox, Emily H. Allen, Matthew C. Keifer *Environmental Health Perspectives*, Vol. 108, No. 6 (Jun., 2000), pp. 515–520

192  Fallon, S. *Nourishing Traditions.* Washington, DC: New Trends; 1999:13-14.

193  Federal Register, 1985.

194  Fallon, Sally, and Mary Enig. "The Great Con-ola." The Weston A. Price Foundation. 28 July 2002. Web. 01 Sept. 2010. <http://www.westonaprice.org/know-your-fats/559-the-great-con-ola.html>.

195  Enig, Mary, and Sally Fallon. "The Skinny on Fats." The Weston A. Price Foundation. 01 Sept. 2001. Web. 02 Sept. 2010. <http://www.westonaprice. org/know-your-fats/526-skinny-on-fats.html>.

196  Mapes, Diane. "Gooey Nutrition Bars Fuel Energy —and Cavities—Health—Oral Health—Msnbc.com." Msnbc. com. Web. 02 Sept. 2010. <http://www.msnbc. msn. com/id/32765018/ns/health-diet_and_ nutrition/>.

197  Brown, E.H & Hansen, R.T The Key to Ultimate Health. Fullerton: Advanced Health Research Publishing; 1998:174.

198  Fallon, S. *Nourishing Traditions.* Washington, DC: New Trends; 1999:51.

199  Huggins, Hal A.. *It's All in Your Head: The Link Between Mercury Amalgams and Illness.* 1 ed. New York: Avery Publishing, 1993. Print:154.

200  Hallberg L, Hulthen L. Prediction of dietary iron absorption: an algorithm for calculating absorption and bioavailability of dietary iron. *Am J Clin Nutr* 2000;71:1147– 60.

201  Bieler, H. *Food is Your Best Medicine.* New York: Vintage Books, 1965: Preface.

202  "Disease, Gum (Diseases, Periodontal)." *ADA: American Dental Association* . N.p., n.d. Web. 16 Sept. 2010. <http://www.ada.org/3063.aspx

203  Price, W. A. *Nutrition and Physical Degeneration* 8th Edition. La Mesa: Price-Pottenger Nutrition Foundation; 2008:506.

204  Ibid. 6th Edition 293.

205  Price, W. A. Nutrition and Physical Degeneration 6th Edition. La Mesa: Price-Pottenger Nutrition Foundation; 2004:290.

206  Vonderplantiz, A. *We Want To Live*: Los Angeles: Carnelian Bay Castle Press;2005: 292. More than five consecutive days of raw eggs may cause thinning of uterine mucus, so a two day break is advised.

207  Radiation Ovens, The Proven Dangers Of Microwaves, Available At: http://www.ecclesia.org/ forum/uploads/bondservant/microwaveP.pdf

208  I. EGLI, L. DAVIDSSON, M.A. JUILLERAT, D. BARCLAY, R.F. HURRELL. "The Influence of Soaking and Germination on the Phytase Activity and Phytic Acid Content of Grains and Seeds Potentially Useful for Complementary Feeding." *Sensory and nutritive qualities of food* 67.9 (2002): 3484-3488. Print.

209  *Am-J. Clin-Nutr.* Baltimore, MD. : American Society for Clinical Nutrition. Jan 1991. V. 53 (1) p. 112-119. Calcium: effect of different amounts on nonheme- and heme-iron absorption in humans.

210  Guyenet, Stephan. "A New Way to Soak Brown Rice." Whole Health Source. N.p., 4 Apr. 2009. Web. 11 Sept. 2010. <http://wholehealthsource.blogspot.com /2009/04/new-way-to-soak-brown-rice.html>.

211  *Stroke.* 2004;35:496.

212  "Oral Health for Older Americans—Fact Sheets and FAQs—Publications—Oral Health." *Centers for Disease Control and Prevention.* N.p., n.d. Web. 16 Sept. 2010. <http://www.cdc.gov/ oralhealth/publications/ factsheets/adult_older.htm>

213  Price, W. A. *Nutrition and Physical Degeneration 6th Edition.* La Mesa: Price-Pottenger Nutrition Foundation; 2004:Chapter 19.

214  Page, M. Abrams, L. *Your Body is Your Best Doctor.* New Canaan: Keats Publishing Inc.;1972:197.

215  Ibid., 197.

216  Price, W. A. *Nutrition and Physical Degeneration 6th Edition.* La Mesa: Price-Pottenger Nutrition Foundation; 2004:337-38.

217  Ibid., 197.

218  Mellanby, Ma. "Periodontal Disease in Dogs (Experimental Gingivitis and "Pyorrhoea")" *Proceedings of the Royal Society of Medicine* April 28, 1930 42-48

219  MELLANBY, EDWARD. *NUTRITION AND DISEASE— THE INTERACTION OF CLINICAL AND EXPERIMENTAL WORK.* London: Oliver and Boyd, 1934. Print.

220  "Client feedback." *Resources for Life.* N.p., n.d. Web. 28 Sept. 2010. <http://www.resourcesforlife.net/ article.asp?article=93>.

221  Phillips , Dr. J.E. . "Dr Phillips Blotting Technique Blotting Brushes" *Seventh Wave Supplements—Additive* Web. 28 Sept. 2010. <http://www.seventhwavesupplements.com/pc/viewPrd.asp?idcategory=107&idproduct=73>

222  Breiner, Mark A.. *Whole-Body Dentistry: Discover The Missing Piece To Better Health.* 1 ed. Fairfield: Quantum Health Press, 1999. Print.

223  Huggins, Hal A.. *It's All in Your Head: The Link Between Mercury Amalgams and Illness.* 1 ed. New York: Avery Publishing, 1993:64. Print.

224  "ATSDR—2007 CERCLA Priority List of Hazardous Substances." *ATSDR Home.* N.p., n.d. Web. 28 Sept. 2010. < http://www.atsdr.cdc.gov/ cercla/07list.html>

225  G Null, M Feldman. "Mercury Dental Amalgams: The Controversy Continues." *Journal of Orthomolecular Medicine*, Vol. 17, No. 2, 2nd Quarter 2002

226  Food and Drug Administration, "Questions and Answers on Amalgam Fillings." www.fda.gov/ cdrh/consumer/amalgams.html. Statement and website was then changed, http://www.fda.gov/ MedicalDevices/ProductsandMedicalProcedures/DentalProducts/DentalAmalgam/ucm171120.htm

227  Principles of Ethics and Code Of Professional Conduct, 2010 American Dental Association <http://www.ada.org/ sections/about/pdfs/ada_code.pdf>

228  Breiner, Mark A.. *Whole-Body Dentistry: Discover The Missing Piece To Better Health.* 1 ed. Fairfield: Quantum Health Press, 1999:70. Print.

229  Ibid.

230  Brown, E.H & Hansen, R.T The Key to Ultimate Health. Fullerton: Advanced Health Research Publishing; 1998:62-63.

231  Huggins, Hal A.. *It's All in Your Head: The Link Between Mercury Amalgams and Illness.* 1 ed. New York: Avery Publishing, 1993:76. Print.

232  Cook, Douglas DDS *Rescued by My Dentist*: 141.

233  Brown, E.H & Hansen, R.T The Key to Ultimate Health. Fullerton: Advanced Health Research Publishing; 1998:89.

234  Huggins, Hal A.. *It's All in Your Head: The Link Between Mercury Amalgams and Illness.* 1 ed. New York: Avery Publishing, 1993:80. Print.

235  Brown, E.H & Hansen, R.T The Key to Ultimate Health. Fullerton: Advanced Health Research Publishing; 1998:78-79.

236  Ibid.

237  Huggins, Hal A.. *It's All in Your Head: The Link Between Mercury Amalgams and Illness.* 1 ed. New York: Avery Publishing, 1993:81. Print.

238  Brown, E.H & Hansen, R.T The Key to Ultimate Health. Fullerton: Advanced Health Research Publishing; 1998:78.

239  Cook, Douglas DDS *Rescued by My Dentist*: 108.

240  Sources were: prlabs.com and nutrimost.net

241  Jones, M. An Interview with George Meinig. Reprinted in *PPNF Journal*, Volume 31, Number 1.

242  Cook, Douglas DDS "Rescued by My Dentist.": 62.

243  Breiner, M. DDS *Whole-Body Dentistry.* Fairfield: Quantum Health Press; 1999:96.

244  Brown, E.H & Hansen, R.T The Key to Ultimate Health. Fullerton: Advanced Health Research Publishing; 1998:105.

245  Gammal, Robert. "Focal Infection in dentistry." *Robert Gammal's Home Page.* N.p., n.d. Web. 23 Sept. 2010. <http:// www.robertgammal.com/ RCTDocs2/FocalInfection.html>.

246  Brown, E.H & Hansen, R.T The Key to Ultimate Health. Fullerton: Advanced Health Research Publishing; 1998:74.

247  Ibid., 76.

248  Cook, Douglas DDS "Rescued by My Dentist.": 125.

249  M.N. Rasool, S. Govender. *THE JOURNAL OF BONE AND JOINT SURGERY*, VOL. 71-B, No. 5, NOVEMBER I989

250  Ibid., 293.

251  H. Wada, H. Tarumi, S. Imazato, M. Narimatsu, and S. Ebisu, "In vitro Estrogenicity of Resin Composites" *J Dent Res* 83(3):222-226, 2004. Available at: http://jdr.iadrjournals.org/ cgi/reprint/83/3/222.pdf

252  Addy, Martin, W Michael Edgar, Graham Embery, and Robin Orchardson. *Tooth Wear and Sensitivity: Clinical Advances in Restorative Dentistry.* 1 ed. Stockholm: Informa Healthcare, 2000:323. Print.

253  Ibid. Ch. 14.

254  "Titanium Dioxide Classified as Possibly Carcinogenic to Humans." CCOHS: Canada's National Centre for Occupational Health and Safety information. N.p., n.d. Web. 29 Sept. 2010. <http://www.ccohs.ca/headlines/ text186.html>.

255  Kumazawa, R. "Effects of Titanium ions and particles on neutrophil function and morphology." *Biomaterials* Volume 23, Issue 17, September 2002, Pages 3757-3764

256  Dr J. Yiamouyiannus Water Fluoridation & Tooth Decay Study, Fluoride 23:pp55-67, 1990.

257  Kennedy, D. "How To Save Your Teeth," Health Action Press. 1993: 141-142.

258  Kumar & Iida. "The Association Between Enamel Fluorosis and Dental Caries in U.S. Schoolchildren," *Journal of the American Dental Association*, July 2009 (Table 1).

259  Connett, Michael. "The Phosphate Fertilizer Industry: An Environmental Overview." *Fluoride Action Network.* N.p., n.d. Web. 29 Sept. 2010 < http://www.fluoridealert.org/phosphate/overview.htm#4>.

260  "NTEU 280 Fluoride." *NTEU 280 Home Page—EPA Headquarters.* N.p., n.d. Web. 29 Sept. 2010. <http://www.nteu280.org/Issues/Fluoride/NTEU280-Fluoride.htm>.

261  McLellan, Helen. "Consumer Health Articles: FLUORIDATION ." *CONSUMER HEALTH.* N.p., n.d. Web. 29 Sept. 2010. <http://www.consumerhealth.org/ articles/display.cfm?ID=19990817225011>.

262  Sibbison, J.b., "More About Fluoride," Lancet, Volume 336, No. 8717, p. 737 (1990).

263  Price, W. A. Nutrition and Physical Degeneration 6th Edition. La Mesa: Price-Pottenger Nutrition Foundation; 2004: op. cit., Chapter 2.

264  op. cit., p. 174.

265  substance P." *Northern California Cranio-facial Diagnostic Center.* N.p., n.d. Web. 30 Sept. 2010. < http:// www.dentalphysician.com/www07/substance_P.html>

266  Jennnings, Dwight. "medparadigm." *Northern California Cranio-facial Diagnostic Center.* N.p., n.d. Web. 30 Sept. 2010. < http://www.dentalphysician.com/ www07/assmedparadigm.html>.

267  Mechanisms of pain arising from the tooth pulp." *School of Clinical Dentistry.* N.p., n.d. Web. 30 Sept. 2010. < http://www.sheffield. ac.uk/dentalschool/research/groups/neuroscience/pain.html>

268  substance P." *Northern California Cranio-facial Diagnostic Center.* N.p., n.d. Web. 30 Sept. 2010. < http:// www.dentalphysician.com/www07/substance_P.html>

269  Jennnings, Dwight. "medparadigm." *Northern California Cranio-facial Diagnostic Center.* N.p., n.d. Web. 30 Sept. 2010. < http://www.dentalphysician.com/ www07/hyperactivity.html >.

270  Roettger, Mark. *Performance Enhancement and Oral Appliances. A supplement to Compendium, Continuing Education in Dentistry.*Aegis Publications, Newtown 2009:4.

271  Dr. Dwight Jennings, <www.dentalphysician.com>

272  Orthodontics—Dr. Brendand C. Stack, *Dr. Stack—TMJ Pain, TMD Pain.* N.p., n.d. Web. 5 Oct. 2010. <http://www.tmjstack.com/ortho.htm>.

273  Jennings, Dwight. "selfassessment." *Northern California Cranio-facial Diagnostic Center.* N.p., n.d. Web. 5 Oct. 2010. < http://www.dentalphysician.com/www07/assselfassessment.html>

274  Mew, John. "Facial Changes in Identical Twins Treated by Different Orthodontic Techniques." *World Journal of Orthodontics* 8.2 (2007): 175-88. Print.

275  Ernst S, Elliot T, Patel A, Sigalas D, Llandro H, Sandy J R and Ireland J. Consent to orthodontic treatment—is it working? *BDJ* 2007. 202:616-617.

276  Kurol,J., Owman-Moll,P and Lundgren,D. 1996. "Time related root resorption after application of a controlled continuous orthodontic force". *American Journal of Orthodontics and Dentofacial Orthopedics.* 110: 303-310.

277  Mohandesan H, Ravanmehr H and Valaei N. 2007. A radiographic analysis of external apical root resorption of maxillary incisors during active orthodontic treatment. *European Journal of Orthodontics* 29: 134-139.

278  Mavragani M, Bfbe O E, Wisth P J and Selvig K A. 2002. Changes in root length during orthodontic treatment: advantages for immature teeth. *European Journal of Orthodontics.* 24: 90-97. 80.

279  Guyenet., Stephan. "Whole Health Source: Malocclusion: Disease of Civilization, Part IX." Whole Health Source. N.p., n.d. Web. 5 Oct. 2010. <http://wholehealthsource. blogspot.com/ 2009/12/malocclusion-disease-of-civilization. html>.

280  Alarashi, M, Franchi, L;Marinelli Andrea, and Defraia B. 2003. Morphometric Analysis of the Transverse Dentoskeletal Features of Class 11 Malocclusion in the Mixed Dentition. *Angle Orthod* 73:21-25.

281  Mew, John. "Facial Changes in Identical Twins Treated by Different Orthodontic Techniques." *World Journal of Orthodontics* 8.2 (2007): 175-88. Print.

282  YouTube ." *Dr John Mew on Dispatches*. N.p., n.d. Web. 3 Oct. 2010. < http://www.youtube.com/watch#!v=pe7OI-PdTno&videos=MDItX4uj6WU&feature=BF>.

283  The craniopath I see, is Dr. Tom Bloink, drbloink.cacranialinstitute.com

284  I have a twin block with a crozat from Dr. Dwight Jennings, www.dentalphysician.com

285  Price, W. A. Nutrition and Physical Degeneration 6th Edition. La Mesa: Price-Pottenger Nutrition Foundation; 2004:288.

286  Ibid., 430.

287  Ibid., 289.

288  Ibid., 64.

289  Ibid. 415.

290  Ibid. 294.

291  op. cit., p. 170.

292  Beltrán-Aguilar, Eugenio D. and Other Authors: Surveillance for Dental Caries, Dental Sealants, Tooth Retention, Edentulism, and Enamel Fluorosis —- United States, 1988—1994 and 1999—2002. Centers for Disease Control and Prevention. Atlanta, 2005. 1-44. 14 Aug. 2007 <http://www.cdc.gov/MMWR/preview/mmwrhtml/ss5403a1.htm>.

293  Anesthesia Morbidity and Mortality, 1988-1999 *Anesth Prog* 48:89-92 2001.

294  Cohen MM, Cameron CB, Duncan PG. "Pediatric Anesthesia Morbidity and Mortality in the Perioperative Period." *Anesthesia & Analgesia* 70 (1990): 160-167. 14 Aug. 2007 <http://www.ncbi.nlm.nih.gov/ sites/entrez?cmd=Retrieve&db=PubMed&list_uids=2301747&dopt=AbstractPlus>. (Original Article Removed from Anesthesia & Analgesia website.)

295  Mellon RD, Simone AF, Rappaport BA."Use of Anesthetic Agents in Neonates and Young Children." Anethsia 104 (2007): 509-520.

296  Berkowitz, Robert J. "Causes, Treatment and Prevention of Early." *Journal of the Canadian Dental Association* 69 (2003): 304-307b. 14 Aug. 2007 <http://www.cda-adc.ca/jcda/vol-69/issue-5/304.pdf>.

297  Huggins, Hal A.. *It's All in Your Head: The Link Between Mercury Amalgams and Illness.* 1 ed. New York: Avery Publishing, 1993:80. Print.

298  Brown, E.H & Hansen, R.T The Key to Ultimate Health. Fullerton: Advanced Health Research Publishing; 1998:78-79.

299  Ibid.

300  Breiner, M. *Whole Body Dentistry*, Quantum Health Press: 1999:137-138.

301  Roberts, Michelle. " 'No proof' for filling baby teeth." BBC News. N.p., n.d. Web. 4 Oct. 2010. <http://news.bbc.co.uk/2/hi/health/8112603.stm>.

302  Ibid.

303  Ibid.

304  Levine, R.S., Pitts, N.B., Nugent, Z.J. "The Fate of 1,587 Unrestored Carious Deciduous Teeth: a Retrospective General Dental Practice Based Study From Northern England." *British Dental Journal* 193 (2002): 99-303. 14 Aug. 2007 <http://www.nature.com/bdj/journal/ v193/n2/full/4801495a.html>.

305  Milsom, K. M., M. Tickle, and D. King. "Does the Dental Profession Know How to Care for the Primary Dentition?" *British Dental Journal* 195 (2003): 301-303. 14 Aug. 2007 <http://www.nature.com/bdj/journal/v195/n6/full/4810525a.html>. Reprinted by permission from Macmillian Publishers LT [*BRITISH DENTAL JOURNAL*] 195 (2003): 301-303.

306  Ibid.

307  Roberts, J.F., Attari, N., Milsom, K. M., M. Tickle, and D. King. "Primary Dentition" *British Dental Journal* 196 (2004): 64-65. 14 Aug. 2007 <http://www.nature.com/bdj/journal/v196/n2/full/4810920a.html>.

308  MELLANBY, EDWARD. *NUTRITION AND DISEASE—THE INTERACTION OF CLINICAL AND EXPERIMENTAL WORK.* London: Oliver And Boyd, 1934. Chapter 11. Print.

309  Breiner, M. *Whole Body Dentistry* Quantum Health Press: 1999:212-213.

310  Ibid., 213

311  Ibid., 86.

312  Ibid., 192.

313  AAP. Breast-feeding and the use of human milk. Pediatrics. 1997;100:1035-1039. <http://www. aapd.org/ members/referencemanual/pdfs/02-03/Breast Feeding.pdf>.

314  Policy on Early Childhood Caries (ECC): Classifications, Consequences, and Preventive Strategies REFERENCE MANUAL V 31 / NO 6 09 / 10 <http://www. aapd.org/media/Policies_ Guidelines/P_ECCClassifications.pdf>.

315  "American Academy of Pediatric Dentistry—Media Information." *PRESS RELEASE: Breastfeeding and Infant Tooth Decay.* Apr. 1999. Web. 06 Oct. 2010. <http://www.aapd.org/media/ pressreleases/breastfeeding-99.asp>.

316  *The Womanly Art of Breastfeeding.* La Leche League International; 2003: 246.

317  Palmer, Brian. «Breastfeeding and Infant Caries.» Brian Palmer, DDS. 14 Aug. 2007 <http://www.brianpalmerdds.com/caries.htm>.

318  "Mouth Breathing—The Root Cause?." *Nose Breathe Mouthpiece: Health Benefits of Nasal Breathing.* N.p., n.d. Web. 6 Oct. 2010. <http://www.nosebreathe. com/mouthbreathing.html>.

# Index

# *NOTES*

## CHAPTER II

[1]Cf. "Scientific Humanism: A Formulation," by Lloyd Morain and Oliver L. Reiser, in the *Humanist*, Vol. III, 1943, pp. 15-19.

## CHAPTER III

*In the writing of the present chapter I have made use of several ideas advanced by Mr. Norman Dodd and Mr. Fritz Kunz of the Guild of American Economists.

[1]The postulates of serial order are stated by the writer in *Philosophy and the Concepts of Modern Science*, pp. 178-79.

[2]These matters are discussed in detail in my two previous studies of the significance of *zero* and $\sqrt{-1}$ for science and philosophy, namely, *A New Earth and a New Humanity*, Chapter VIII, and *Planetary Democracy* (with Blodwen Davies), Chapters XI and XII. An understanding of the place of these in our thinking is essential to a full understanding of the argument in the present book.

[3]Cf. "Science As International Humanism," *Humanist*, Summer, 1943.

## CHAPTER IV

[1]Cf. "The Work of Dr. C. Hilton Rice in Extra-Sensory Perception," by Dr. J. G. Pratt, *Journal of Parapsychology*, 1937, Vol. I, 239-259.

[1]This was a decade ago. Within the last several years I have received a letter from Dr. S. Howard Bartley of the Laboratory of Neurophysiology at Washington University (St. Louis), an expert in the field of vision who has been investigating the afferent side of vision. Now it turns out that Dr. Bartley seems to be thinking along lines which would be welcomed by Dr. Rice as tending to confirm some of his own speculation on the visual reaction arc. I quote from Dr. Bartley's letter: "I have shifted over temporarily from the afferent side to the motor side, and am investigating pupil behavior. The pupil in its action seems to parallel quantitatively certain features of brightness discrimination. For example, if a bright disc in a dark field were presented to one eye the pupil would constrict as the intensity of the disc is increased. If one adds another disc alongside the first one while the second one is still dim, the pupil dilates. As the intensity of the second disc is raised to match that of the first, the pupil again constricts. The parallel to this in brightness discrimination is the fact that the bright disc looks brighter before the second disc was inserted alongside of it. It was dimmed, you see, by the presence of the second disc, but when the latter was raised in intensity to equal the first disc the two look brighter than the single disc. The total flux from the two is

similarly now able to constrict the pupil beyond what it was with a single disc. Other examples similar in principle can be cited to show that when the observer "sees" a surface of an object as dim, regardless of its intrinsic intensity, the pupil is larger than when he "sees" it as bright. Thus what has ordinarily been thought of as a "simple" reflex is quite like sensation in its capers."

The moral of this tale, as I interpret it, is that the old-fashioned neurology of the one-way reflex arc is entirely inadequate. Needless to say, Dr. Bartley's views are not cited as verification of Dr. Rice's ESP speculations. [Footnote by O.L.R.]

[2]Gestalt theory recognizes this when it employs the notion of an *attraction of forces* in the underlying brain processes to explain certain facts of perceptual ("phenomenal") patterns. Thus two parts of the brain which are structurally distinct may, in terms of energy-coordinates, be functionally "closer" together than two areas which are separated by a smaller spatial interval. This explanation of Wertheimer's *phi-phenomenon* —the production of "seen" motion through a process of short-circuiting in the brain—has a parallel in electrodynamics in the attraction of two parallel conductors for each other when currents are flowing through them.

[3]Einstein and Infeld, *The Evolution of Physics,* p. 158; also pp. 255-260 and 310-314.

[4]Cf. "Foundations of Mathematical Biophysics," *Philosophy of Science,* 1934, Vol. I, 176-196; and "On the Physical Nature of 'Cytotropism,'" *J. Gen. Physiol.,* 1932, Vol. 15, 298-306.

[5]On this point see A. J. Lotka's *Elements of Physical Biology,* 1925, p. 76.

[6]This important fact was first pointed out to me by Prof. William M. Martin of the University of North Carolina (Women's College).

[7]Cf. "The Beginnings of Social Behavior in Unicellular Organisms," by H. S. Jennings, *Science,* 1940, Vol. 92, Dec. 13.

[8]This idea is developed in our book, *A New Earth and a New Humanity,* 1942, Chapter IX.

[9]See his very interesting article, "Mind and Matter," *Journal of the American Society for Psychical Research,* 1942, Vol. 36, 113-121.

[10]Cf. "Haunting and the 'Psychic Ether' Hypothesis; With Some Preliminary Reflections on the Present Conditions and Possible Future of Psychical Research,.. by H. H. Price. *Proceedings of the Society for Psychical Research,* Dec., 1939 (Vol. XLV), 307-343.

[11]For a fuller discussion of this idea see the author's books, *Philosophy and the Concepts of Modern Science,* pp. 168-169 and *The Promise of Scientific Humanism,* p. 316.

## CHAPTER V

*The present chapter first appeared in *Free World,* October, 1944, and is here reprinted by permission.

## CHAPTER VI

[1]Cf. *Philosophy and the Concepts of Modern Science,* 1935, Ch. XIII; *The Promise of Scientific Humanism,* 1940, Ch. XIX.

[2]In a remarkable article on "The Structure of the Unconscious," in the volume, *The Unconscious; A Symposium,* Kurt Koffka has this to say: "It is . . . probable that the dreamer does know what his dream means, *but does not know that he knows, and therefore believes he does not know.*"

[3]When I first began to speculate in terms of a cortico-thalamic integration (as the basis for what was metaphorically called the head-heart synthesis), I made use of Alfred Korzybski's scheme as presented in his book, *Science and Sanity.* More recently I have come across the volume, *The Neural Basis of Thought,* by George G. Campion and G. Elliott Smith, which develops a theory of the "thalamo-cortical circulation of neural impulses." Prior to my familiarity with both of these sources, however, I had already presented a theory along somewhat similar lines in an article on "The Biological Origins of Religion," in the *Psychoanalytical Review,* January, 1932, Vol. 19.

*This chapter was first published as an article in PHILOSOPHY OF SCIENCE, April 1945, and is herewith republished, with minor changes, with the editor's permission.

CPSIA information can be obtained
at www.ICGtesting.com
Printed in the USA
LVHW030834150223
739355LV00007B/992